THE ART OF

African American Hair Design

also featuring caucasian

by Pamela Berry

The Art of Hair Design
Copyright © 2005-2006 Pamela Berry
All rights reserved. This publication may not be reproduced or quoted in whole or in part in printed or electronic form, or used in presentations on radio, television, videotape, film or other electronic means without written permission from Pamela Bannister Berry Inc.

Written, and photography by Pamela B. Berry
ISBN: 1-4196-0406-6

Publishing at:
BookSurge, LLC
1-866-308-6235

Printed in the United State of America

Interior arrangement/formatting and cover by
Kathrine Rend - Rend Graphics
www.rendgraphics.com

To order additional copies, please contact:
Pamela Berry
1-843-276-1304
E-mail: pbannister@sc.rr.com

Acknowledgements

Although I am given credit for writing this book, the job could never have been completed without the help of so many others. It is imperative that I express my sincere thanks to each person that was a part of this accomplishment.

Special thanks go to Katina Chisholm and Endia President. Also to the staff, directors and students at Charleston Cosmetology Institute. Mr. Poer, a lecturer, consultant, educator, and platform artist has been a big inspiration to me. The opportunity to teach at this school has been very rewarding.

My clients also play an important role throughout my journey to success. Without them, there would be no "ME." It is because of them that I am motivated to develop new styles and techniques in order to continuously provide them with customer satisfaction.

Last, but definitely not least, very special thanks to my husband, my biggest supporter, Quinten Berry. He, along with my family and friends, give me the encouragement I need in order to make my journey to success a little easier. He constantly reminds me that "In Christ, we can do all things." I take pride in saying that he is always by my side.

Thanks to all who helped to make this book possible.

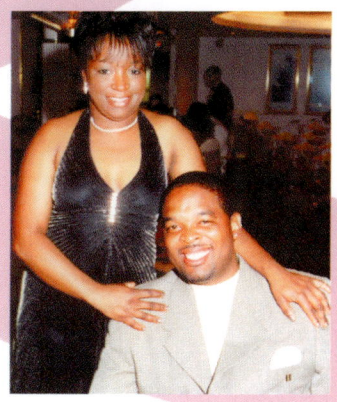

Table of Contents

Chapter One - Rolls 1
- French Roll 2-3
- Classical Bun 4-5
- Artistic Dobby Wrap with rollers 6-7
- Designer Flat Wrap 8-9

Chapter Two - Ponytails 11
- Create a Ponytail with human hair 12-13
- Windmill 14-17
- Loops 18-19
- Bun with pleats 20-23
- Barrel curl with pin curl 24-27
- Stacked pin curl 28-31

Chapter Three - Twist, Coils & Fingerwaves 33
- Fingerwave with curls 34-35
- Flat Twist with water falls 36-37
- Flat Twist with weave 38-39

Chapter Four - Thermal Styling 41
- Press & Curl 42-43
- Marcel Curling Iron 44-45
- Basket Weave Design 46-49

Table of Contents

Chapter Five - Braiding & Extensions — 51
- Single Braids "Off the Scalp Braid" — 52-53
- Silky locks "Dreads" — 54-57
- Cornrow Braiding "On the Scalp Braid" — 58-61

Chapter Six - Weaving — 63
- Hair Extension—Sewing Method — 64-66
- Hair Extension—Bonding Method — 68-69
- Quick Weave Design — 70-71

Foreword

The Art of African American Hair Design is exciting and adventurous in the field of cosmotology. This manual allows you to be creative and illusional in the styling process. Each chapter will teach you how to create a beautiful masterpiece. By learning these concepts and techniques, you will be better equiped to create your own beautiful hair designs!

Due to the use of hair fillers, bobby pins, and rubber bands, etc., special precautions are recommended. Always follow the guide lines of sanitation, sterilization, and the rules of regulation.

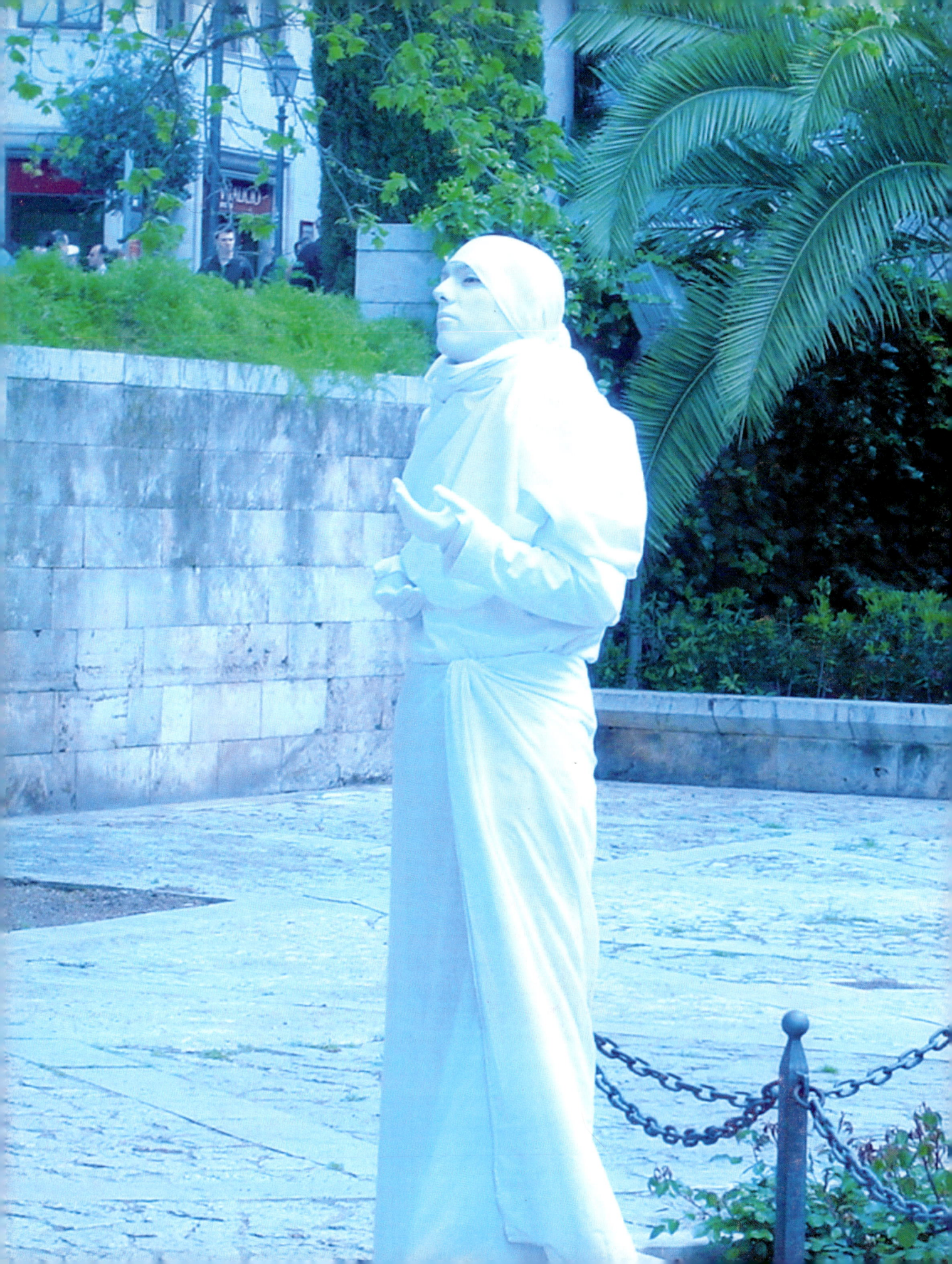

Chapter One

Rolls, Buns & Wraps

Rolls, Buns & Wraps

French Roll

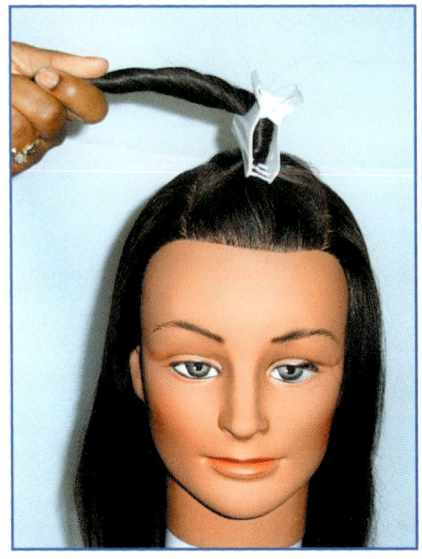

1. Carve out a rectangle from the base of the head, secure with a jaw clip.

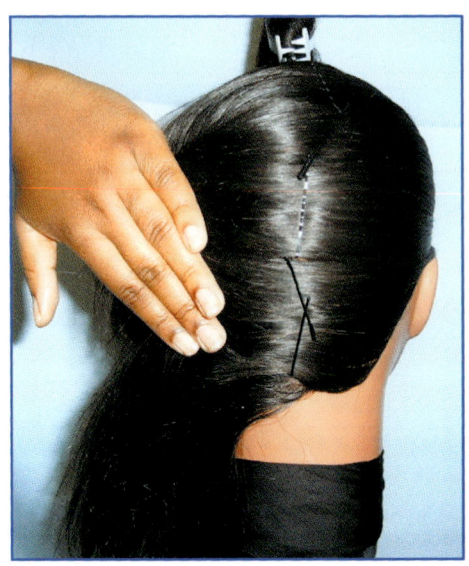

2. Mold hair to the left side of the head and place bobby pins to secure in place.

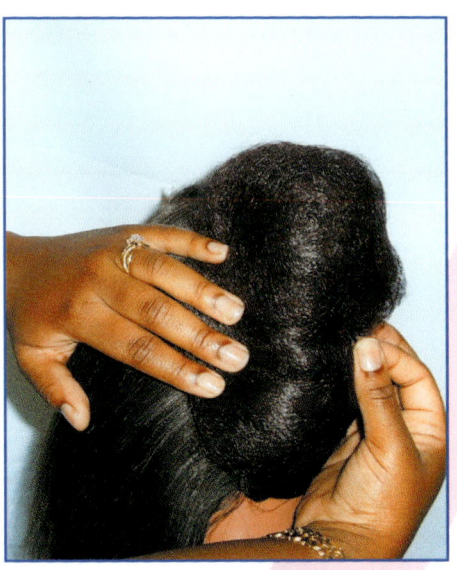

3. Place hair filler on top of bobby pins and secure filler with hair pins to hold in place.

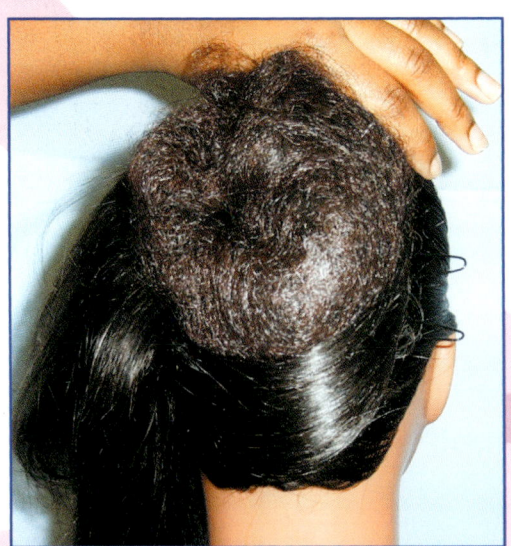

4. Overlap small sections of hair over filler and secure with hair pins.

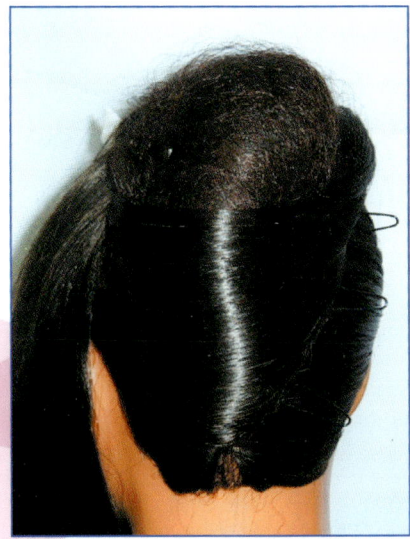

5. Continue to overlap until hair filler is completely covered as you work towards the crown area.

Rolls, Buns & Wraps

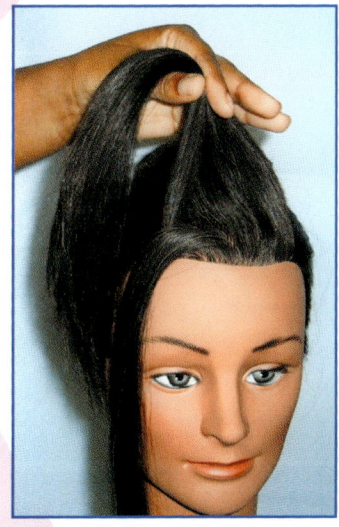
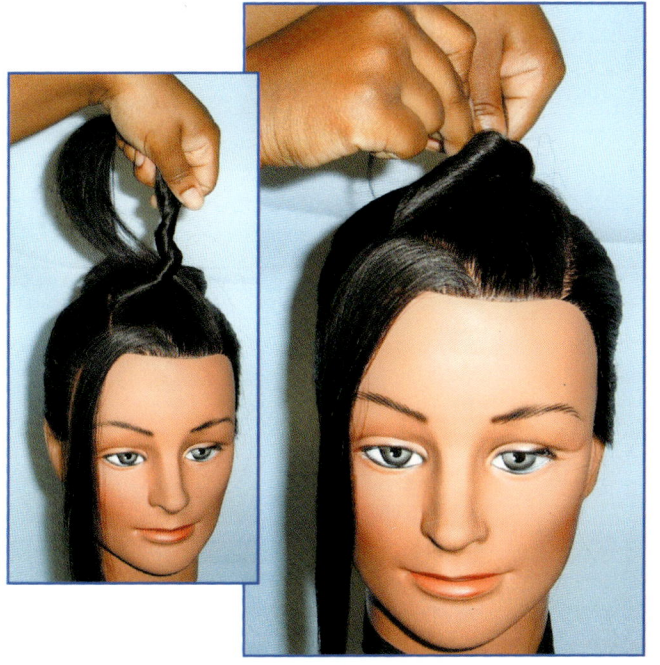
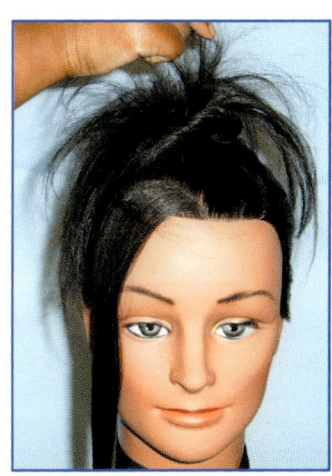

6. Remove clip from rectangle at the top of the head, leaving a small portion to enhance the style.

7. Twist remaining hair strands and secure with hair pins.

8. Fan hair with tail comb or fingers to balance and complete the style.

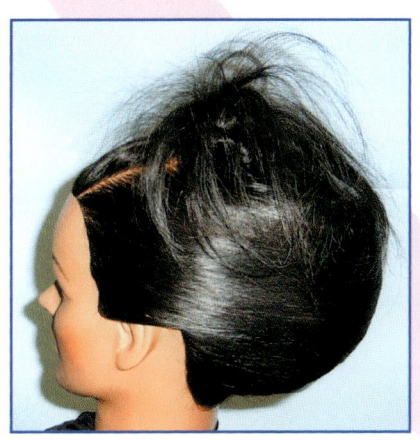

9. Style is complete with a little class!

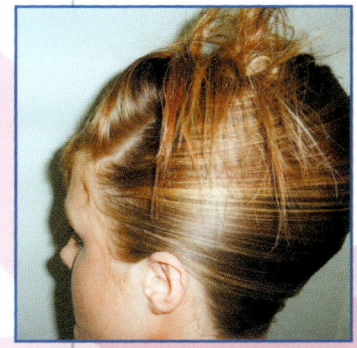
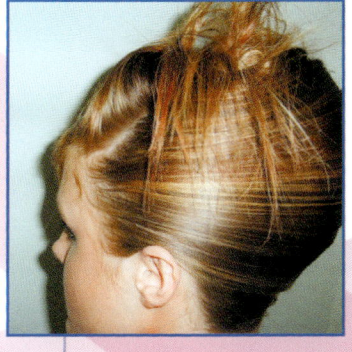

live model

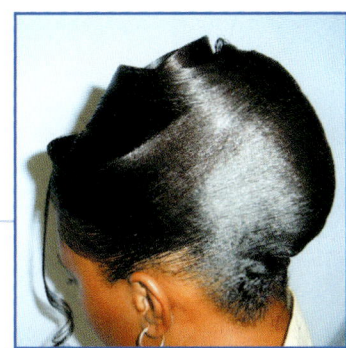

Another variation

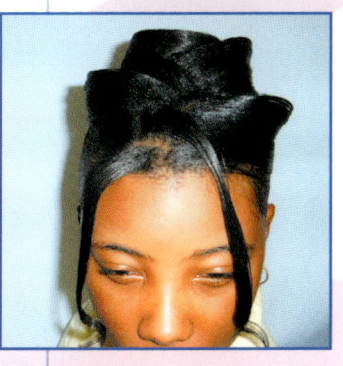

Rolls, Buns & Wraps

Classical Bun

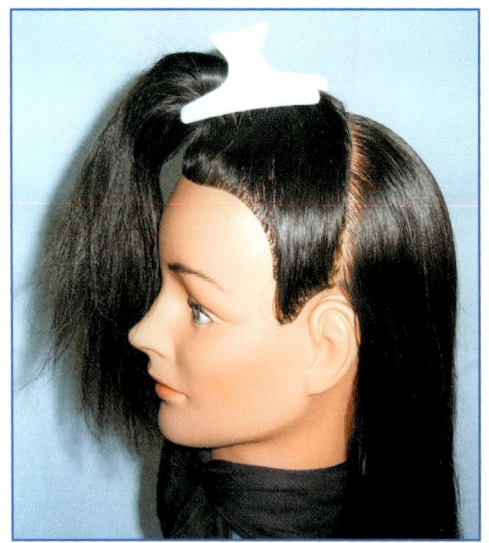

1. Begin by sectioning hair out from ear to ear. Secure crown area with a jaw clip.

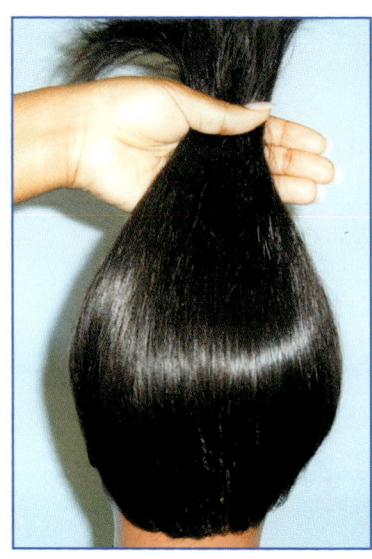

2. The exterior is then molded in an upright position.

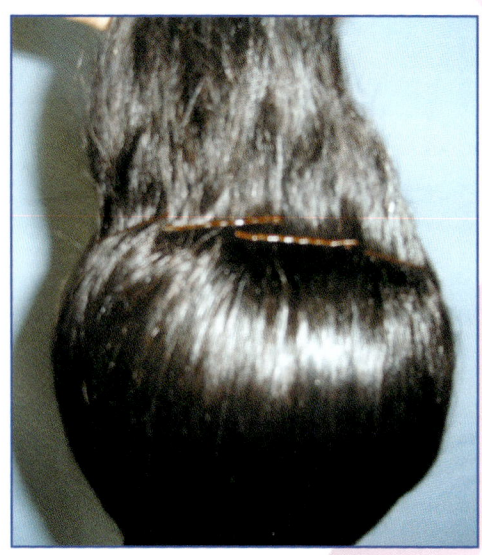

3. Place bobby pins in a horizontal position across the crown area—this should secure the hair in place.

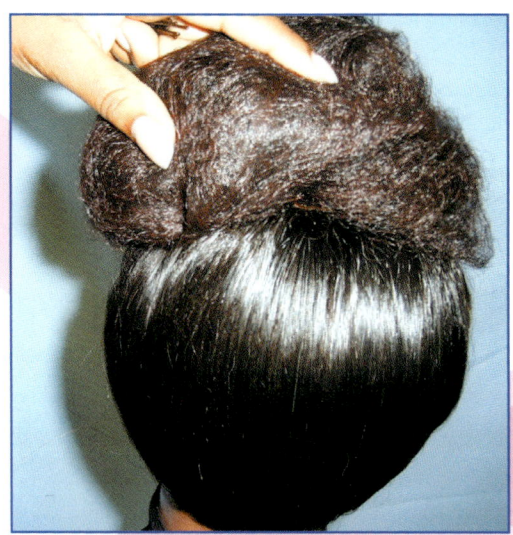

4. Hair filler is then placed on top of the bobby pins and secured. This creates a cushion for the bun.

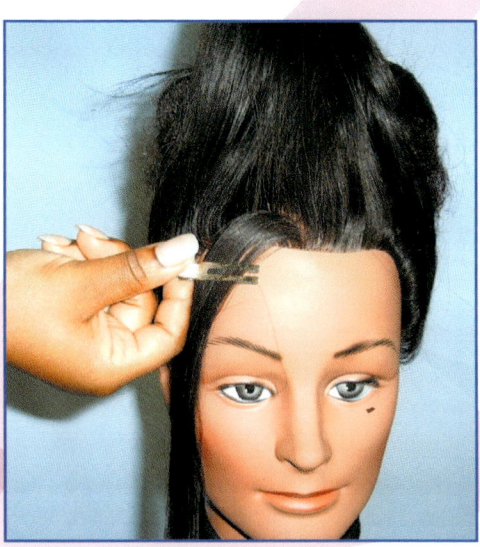

5. Carve out a small section in front. To enhance the design, the remaining hair is blended with hair that was pulled up from the exterior.

Rolls, Buns & Wraps

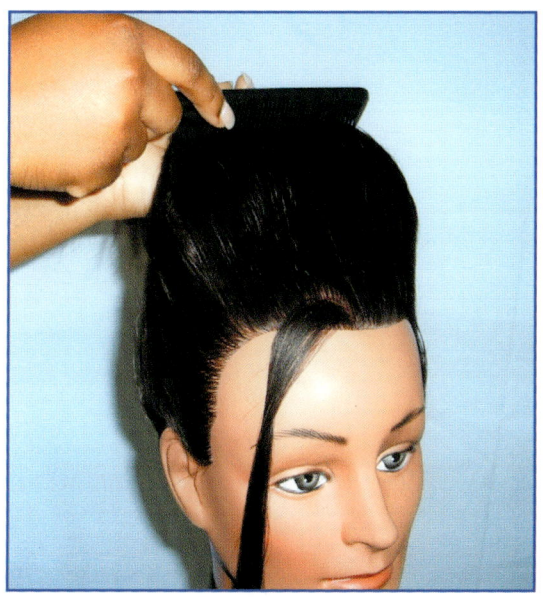

6. Comb hair over filler, to create a smooth appearance.

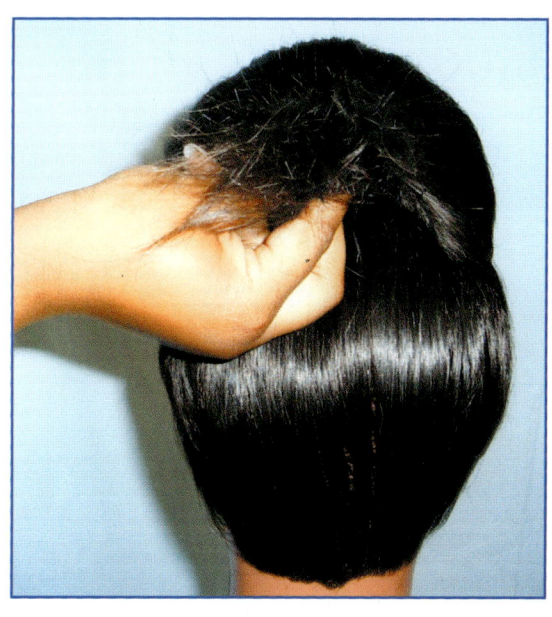

7. Twist ends of hair and secure with hair pins.

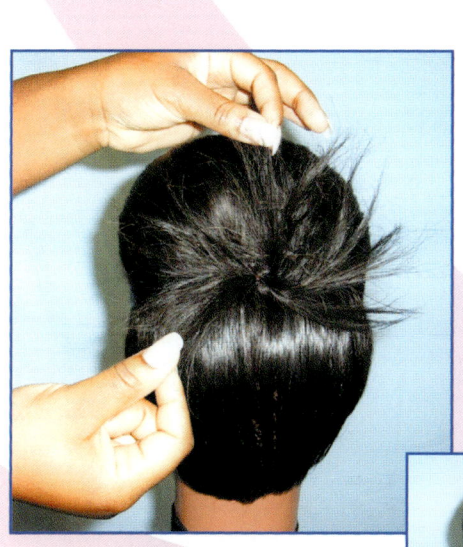

8. Creating a fantail design for this classical bun establishes a more settled look.

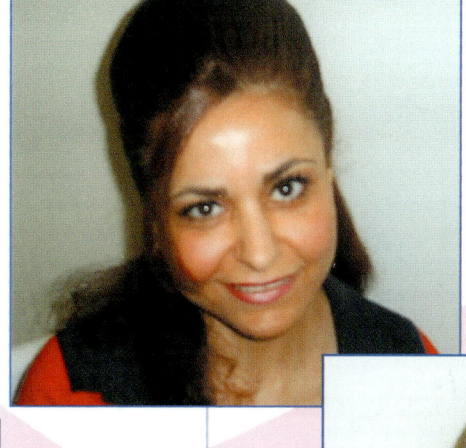

live model

Pin curls or ornamentation could be added to the back of this design

Rolls, Buns & Wraps

Artistic Dobby Wrap
with rollers

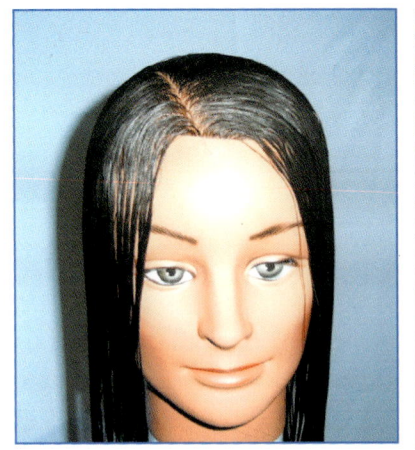

1. Large rollers are used for this design. Begin by making a side part starting from the front hairline.

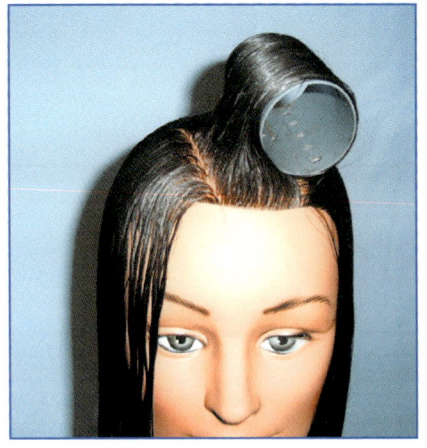

2. The first roller is carved out diameter size of roller and then placed horizontal to the part.

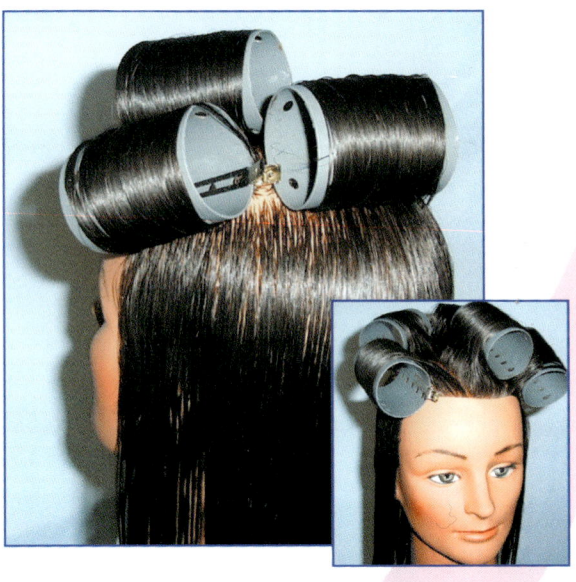

3. Continue to place rollers around the first roller in a circular pattern.

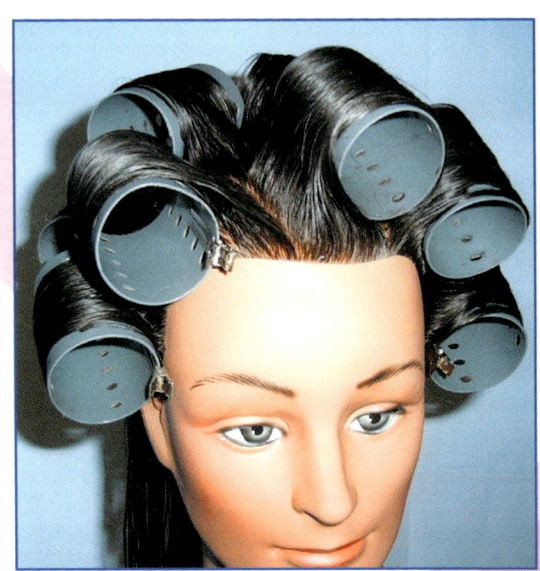

4. Hair should be wrapped around roller with tension. Balancing rollers is very important in order to achieve the best curl pattern.

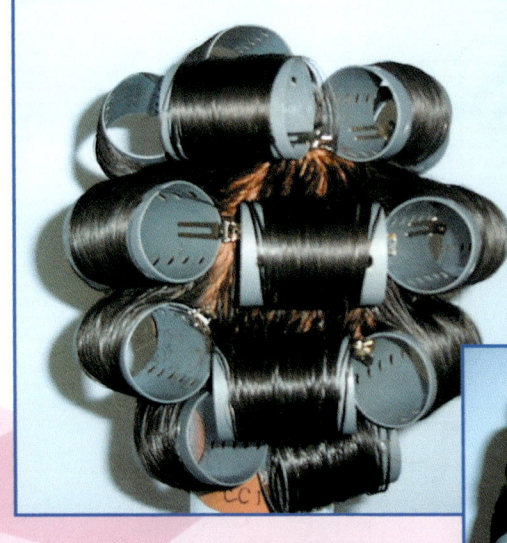

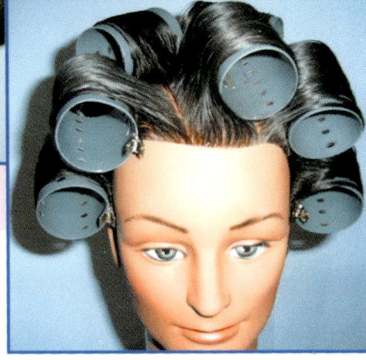

5. Set is dried for thirty to forty-five minutes depending on hair texture.

Rolls, Buns & Wraps

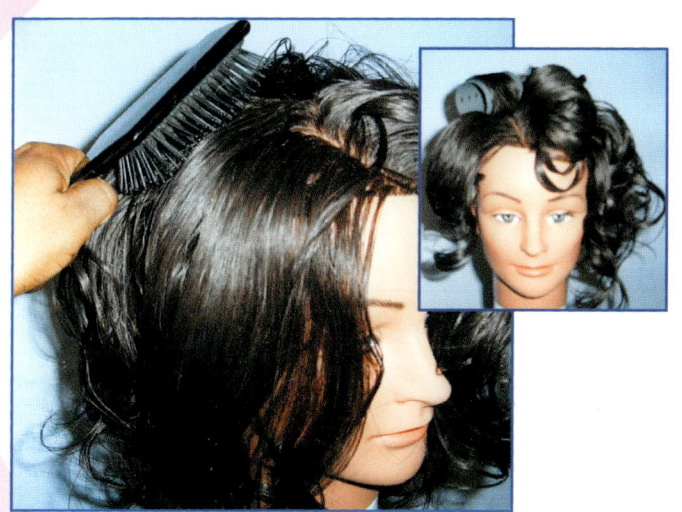

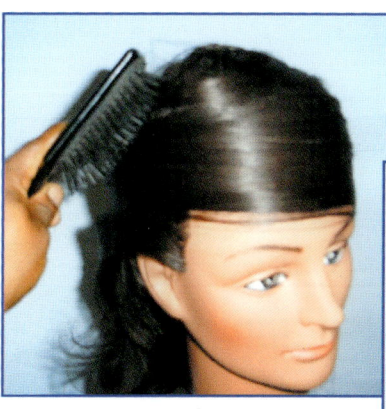

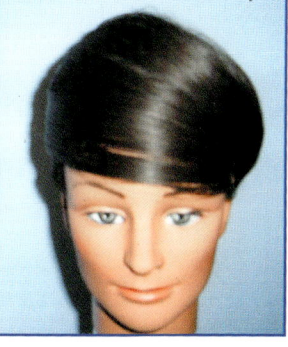

6. Remove rollers and relax curl pattern.

7. Set is then wrapped in a circular pattern. This technique is designed to loosen curl pattern and create body.

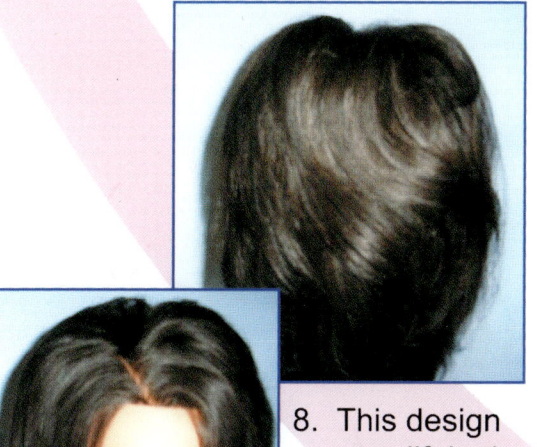

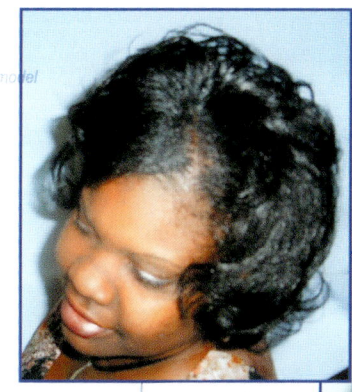

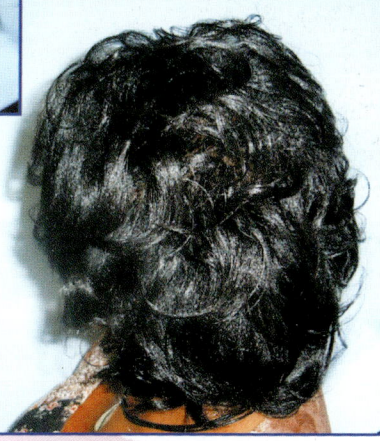

8. This design creates lift in the crown area and bounce around the form.

To create and style with rollers, you must know all positions of roller control that could be used in any particular roller set. Knowledge of roller setting creates good results. Hair in each roller should be the diameter of the base size. This will give a much tighter curl at the base. Without base control, you will end up with a loose curl. Starting a basic roller set in crown area will give you control of the hair.

Rolls, Buns & Wraps

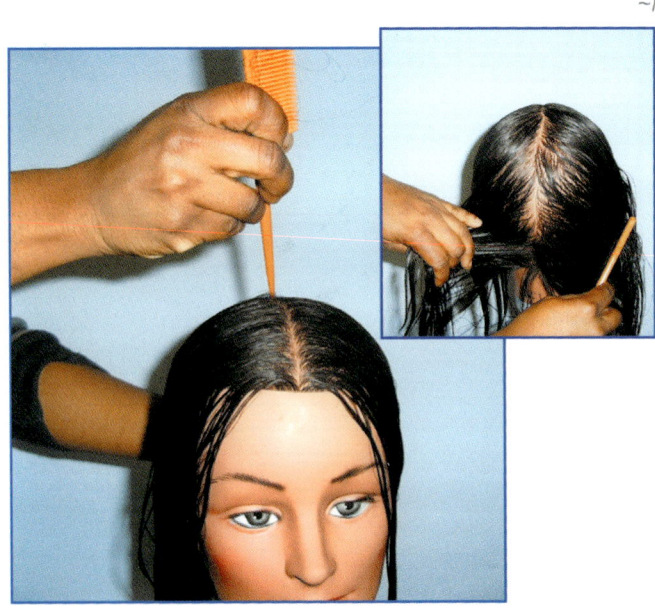

1. Starting at the front hairline. Divide the hair in half from front to nape.

~Hair is shampooed and clean.~

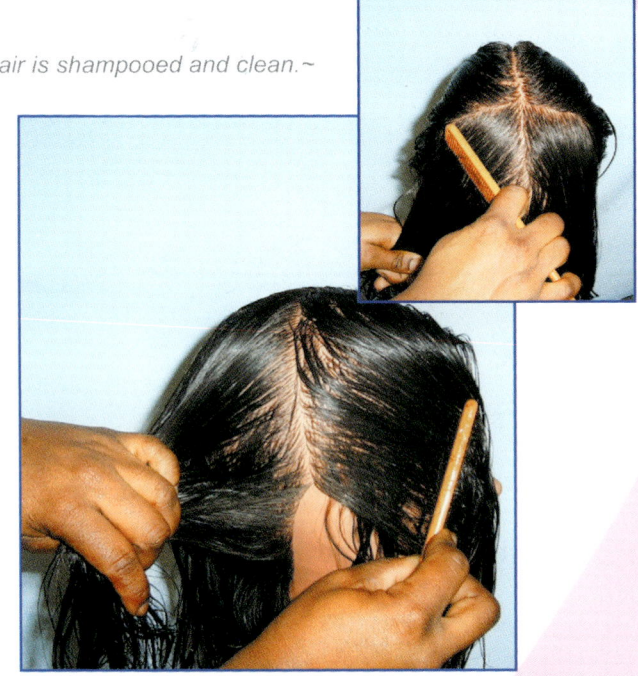

2. Continue to section out from ear to ear. This will give you control of the hair during the wrapping procedure.

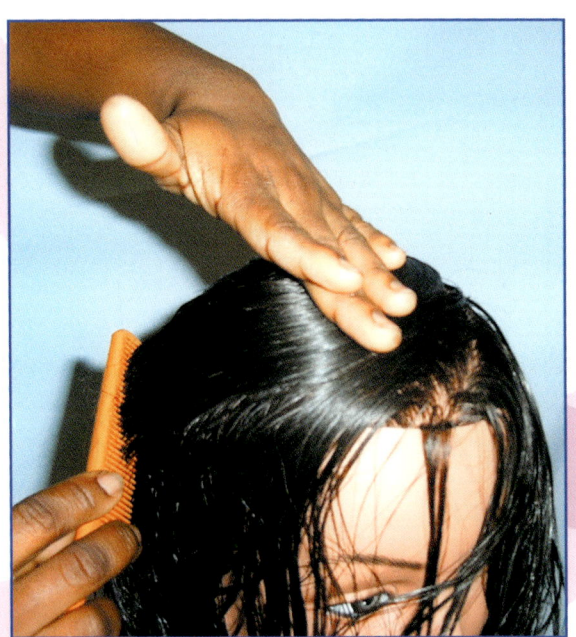

3. Starting directly in the crown area, create a small circle pattern.

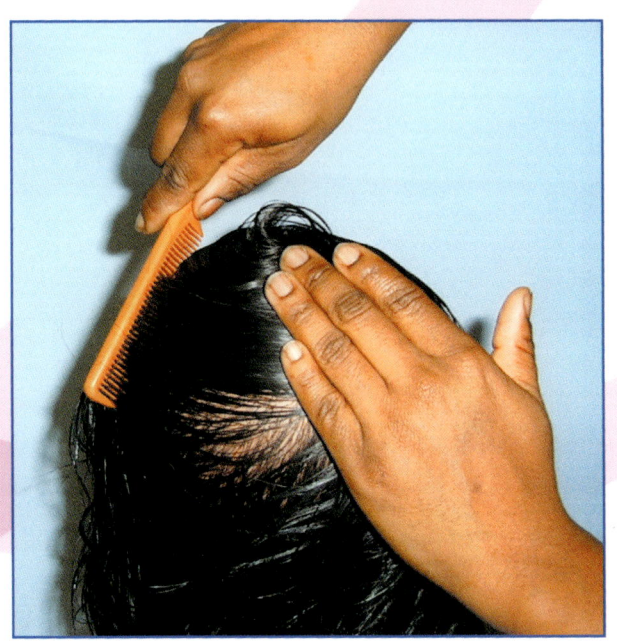

4. Two inches of hair is molded in a circle.

Rolls, Buns & Wraps

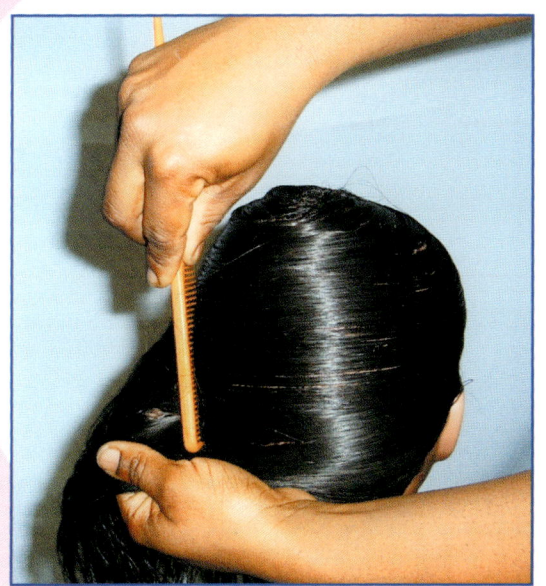

5. Continue to mold hair around the head.

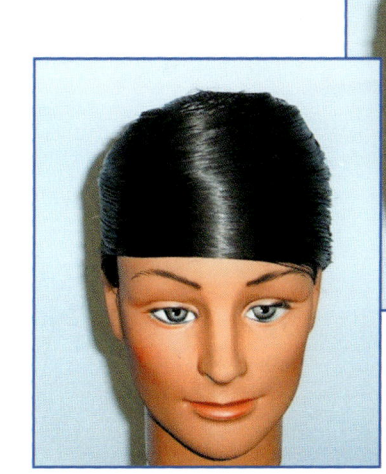

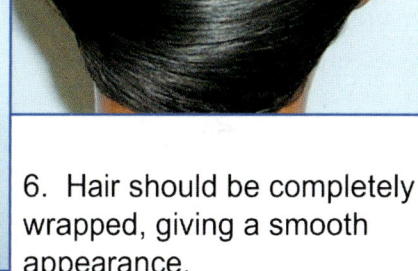

6. Hair should be completely wrapped, giving a smooth appearance.

7. This wet style is placed under the dryer for thirty to forty minutes, depending on the hair texture. Hair is dried completely.

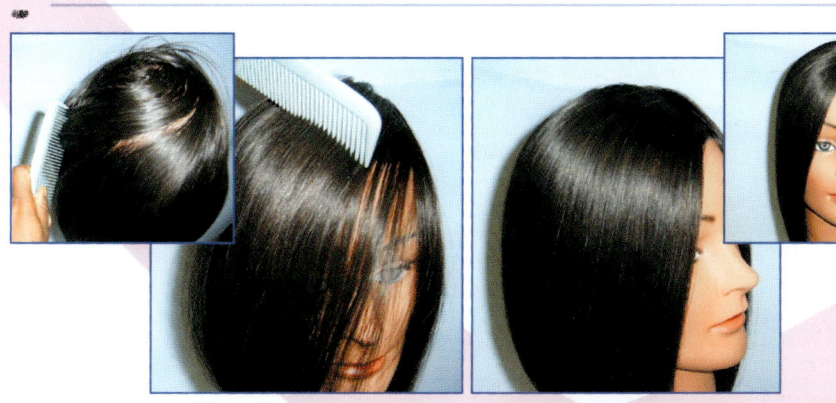

8. Once dried, comb or brush hair out in the pattern it was molded in.

9. This design contours the curve of the head with style.

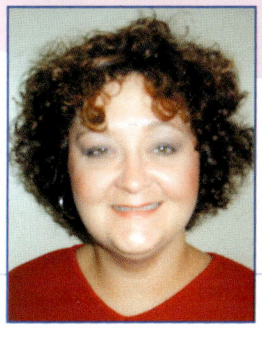
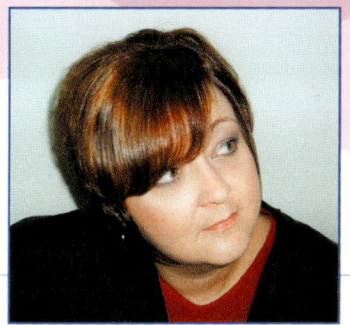
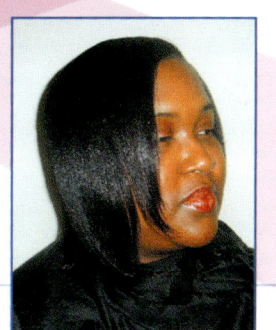

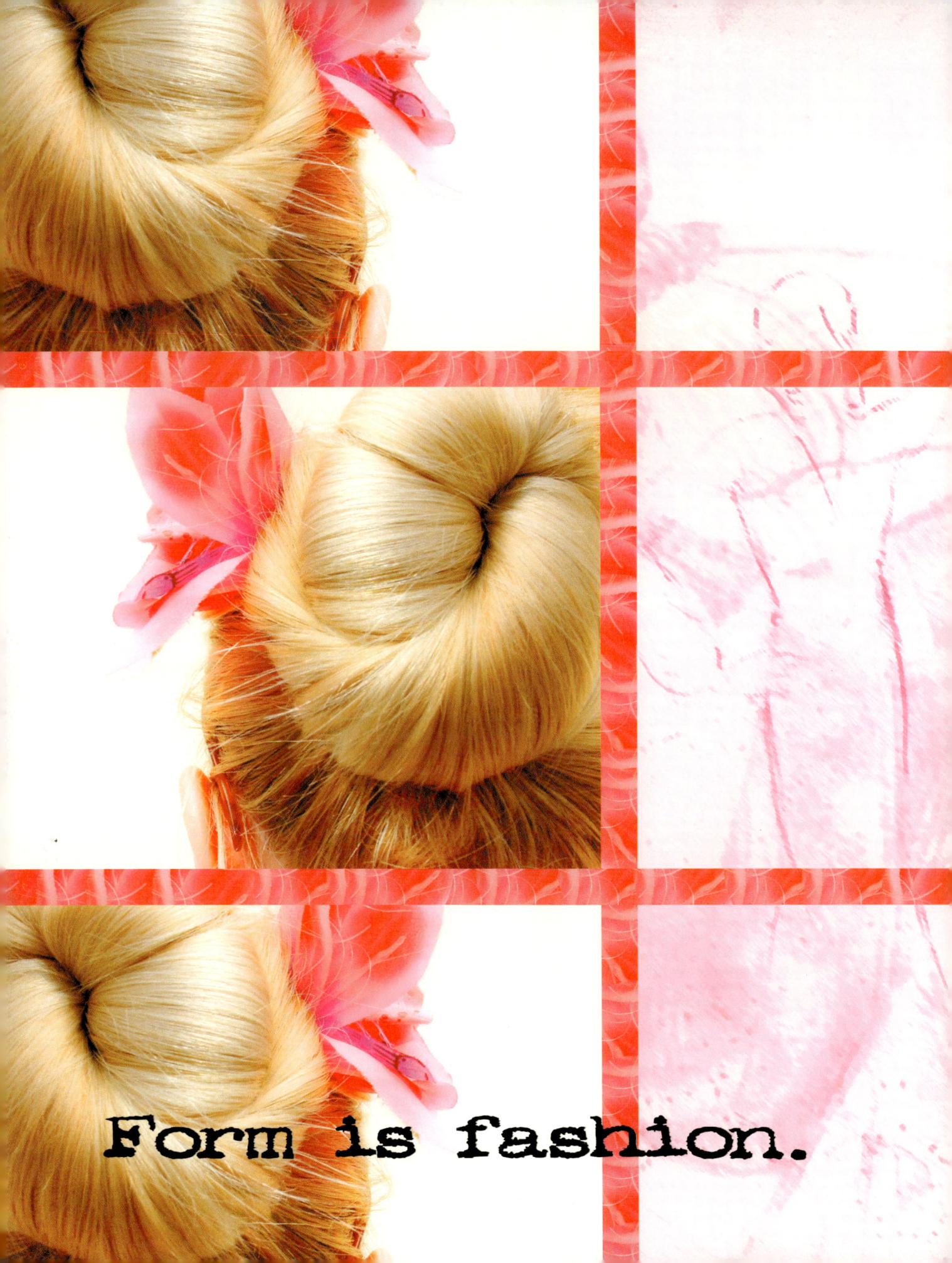

Chapter Two

Ponytails

2

Ponytails

Create a Ponytail
with human hair

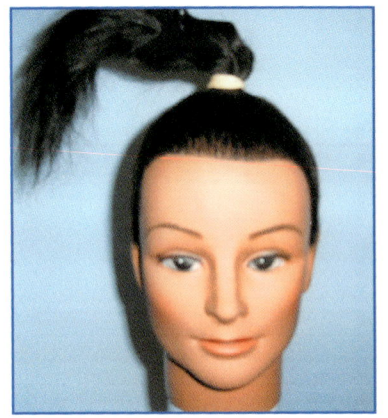
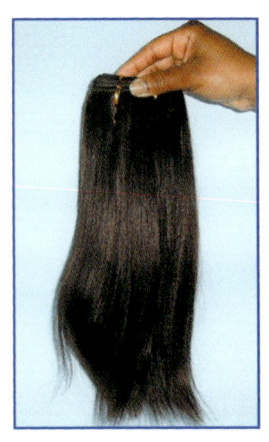

1. Start by placing the natural hair into a ponytail in the crown area. Secure tightly with a rubber band. A 12-inch human hair ponytail is needed.

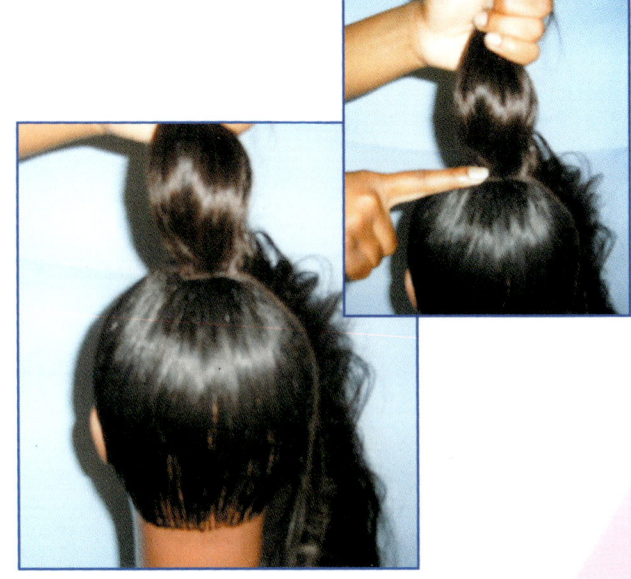

2. Place the weave ponytail hair in an upright position. Secure hair pin at the base of the ponytail. Make sure the base is secured tightly.

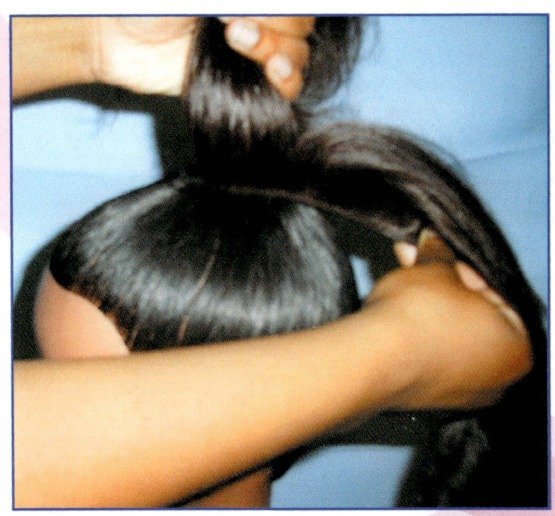

3. During the wrapping procedure, continue to wrap and place hair pins around the base. Make sure hair pins are not placed on the scalp.

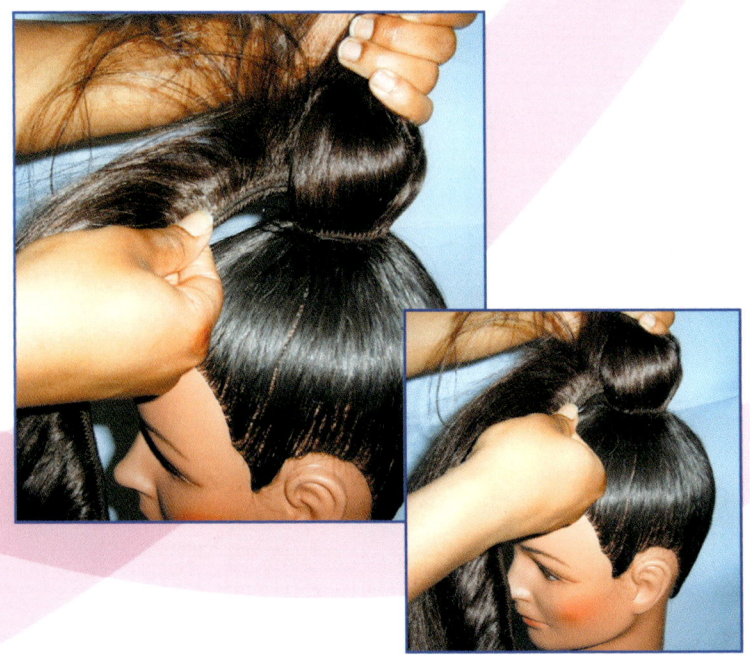

4. The weft of the hair should be wrapped tightly at the base. This will keep the track from lifting.

Ponytails

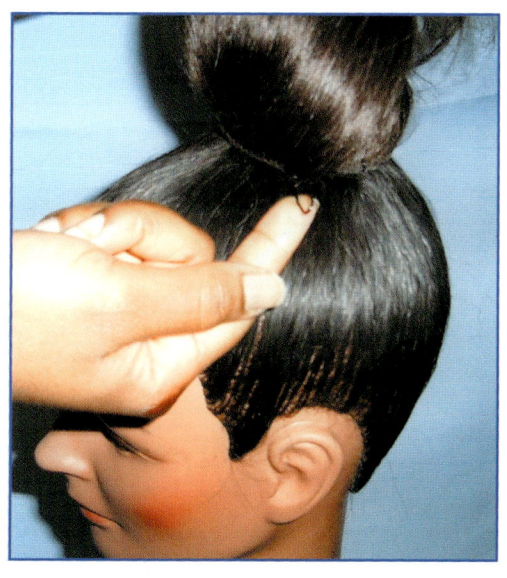

5. Secure the hair pins to close the ponytail at the end of the wrapping procedure.

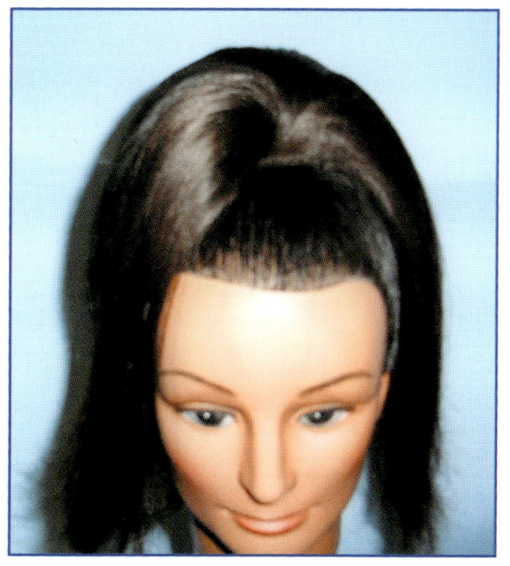

6. A weave ponytail is achieved.

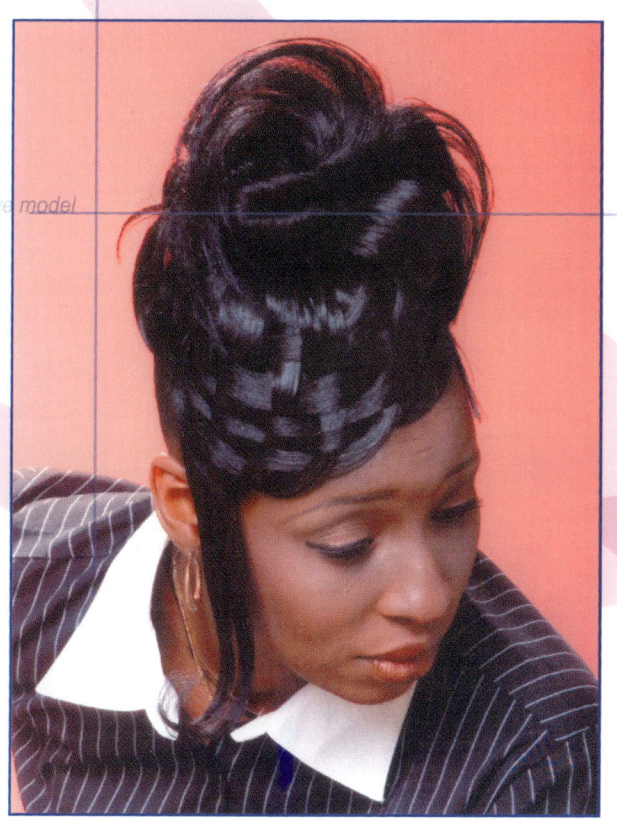

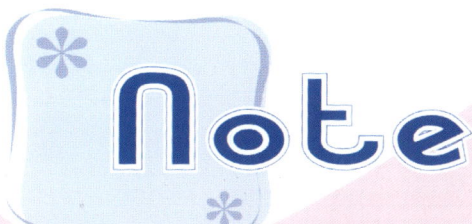

During this chapter you will create different designer ponytails using the technique shown. Each design will provide you with the opportunity to create a hairstyle that is truly unique.

Creativity is everything.

Ponytails

Windmill

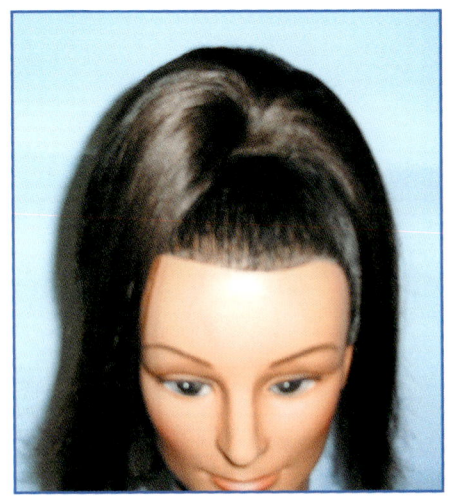
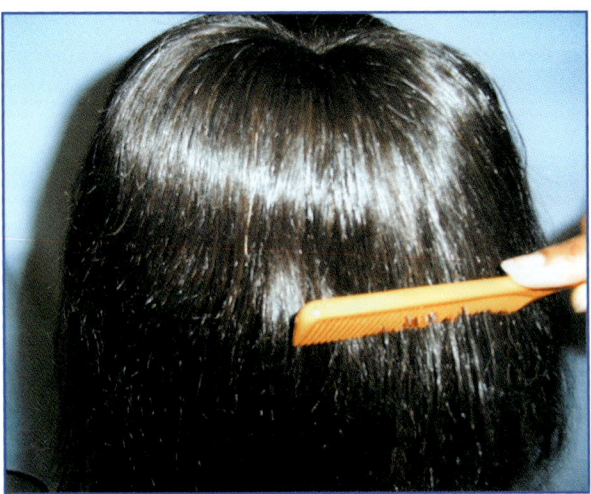

1. Starting with a weave ponytail, mold hair straight down and around the head.

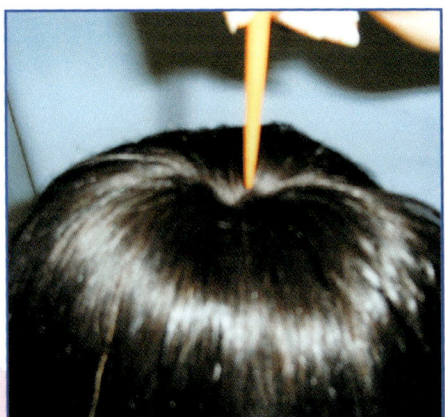
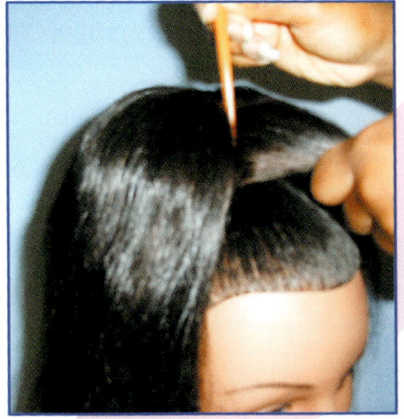

2. From the point of origin, which is the beginning of the design, using a vertical line, section out a two inch subsection.

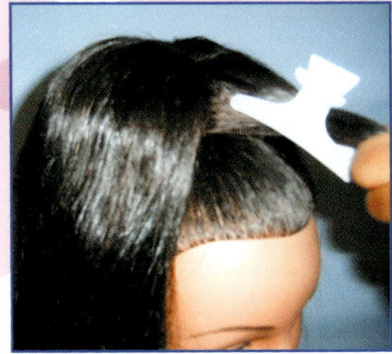

3. Secure with jaw clip, for control.

Ponytails

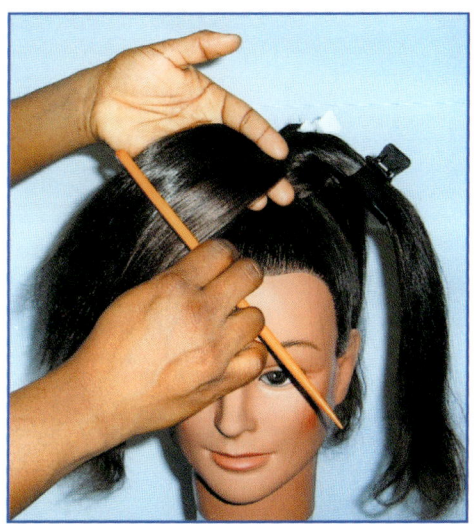

4. Continue to subdivide hair into five or six sections.

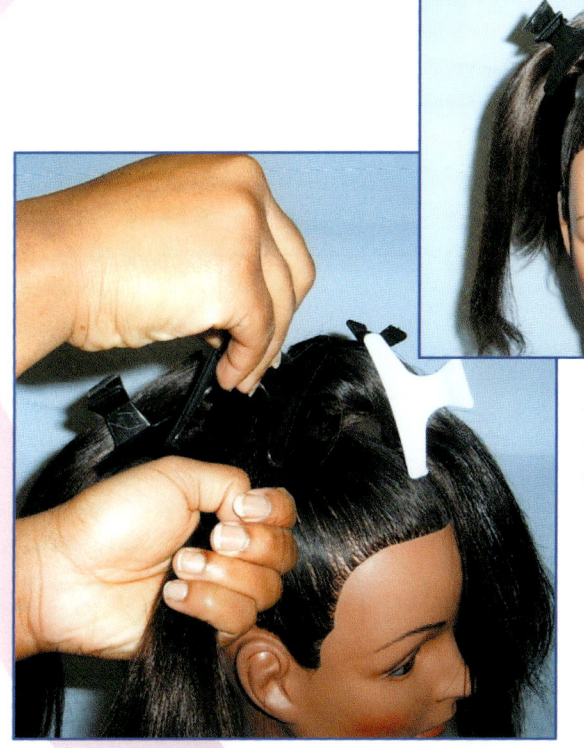

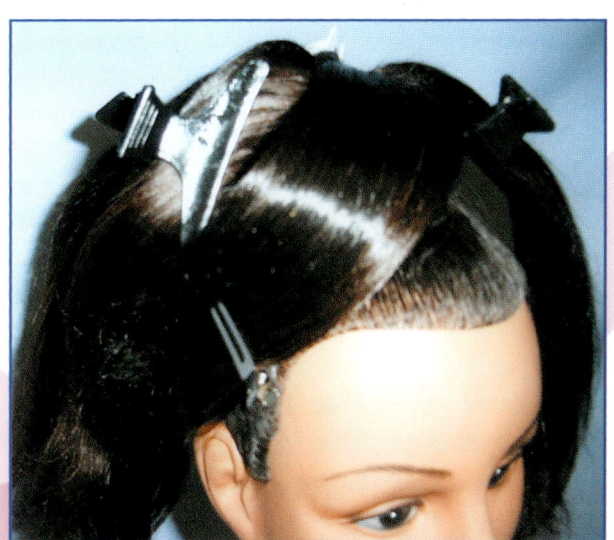

5. Begin the design with the center section closest to the forehead.

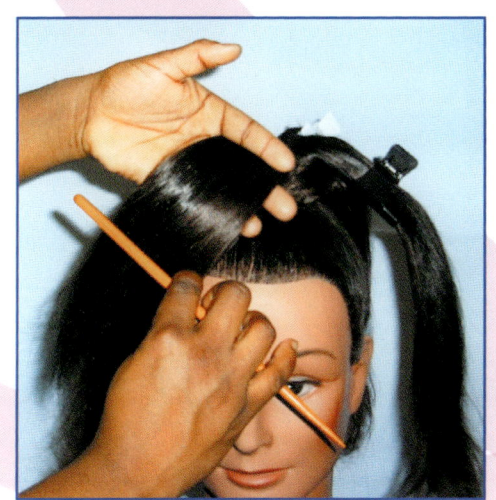

6. Mold hair in a clockwise direction.

7. Place roller clip to hold hair firmly against the head.

15

Ponytails

Windmill
...continued

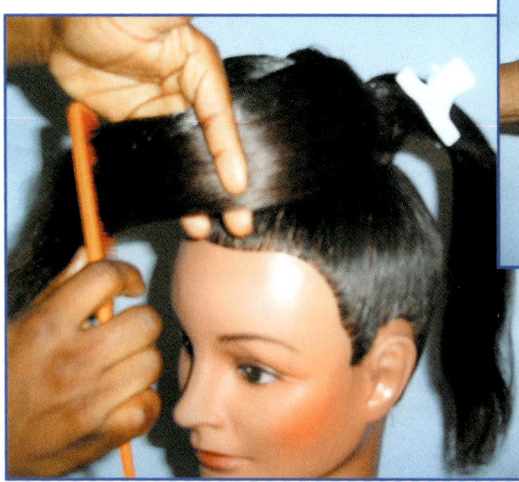
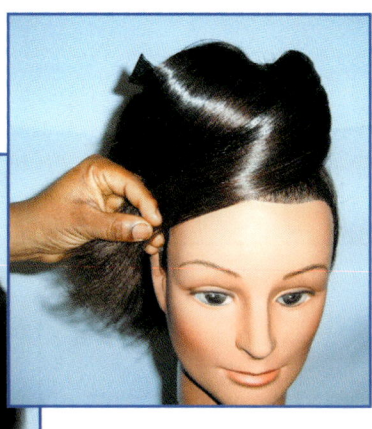

8. Continue to take sections from the counter clockwise direction and mold hair strands in the clockwise direction.

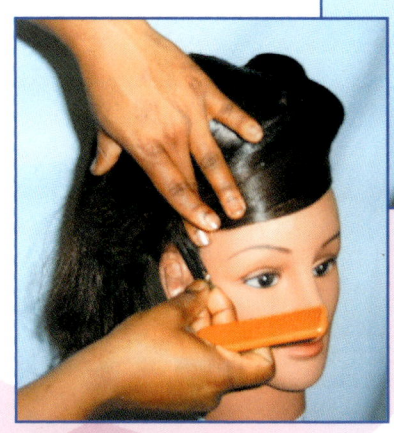

9. Blend hair strands together and clip for control.

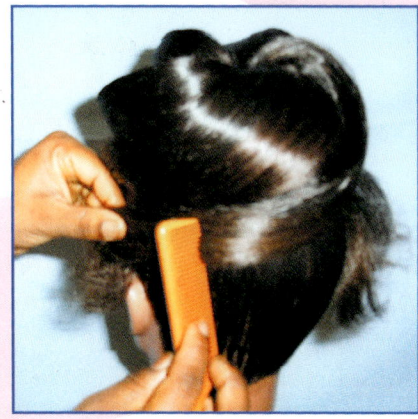

10. Blend last subsection around the previous strand. Remove roller clips. Styling spray is used at this time to set the style.

Ponytails

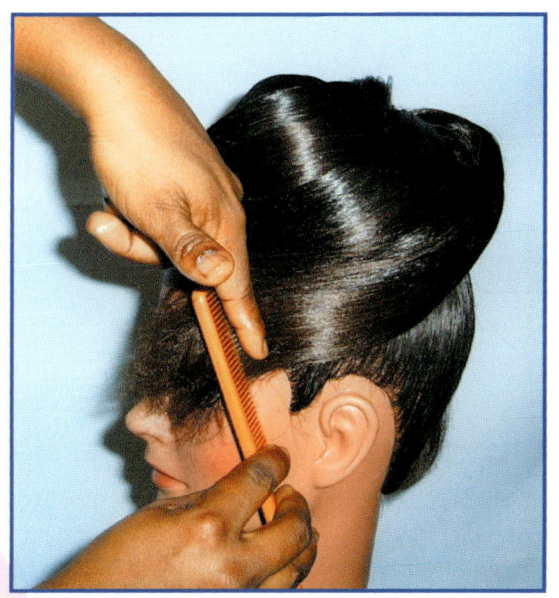
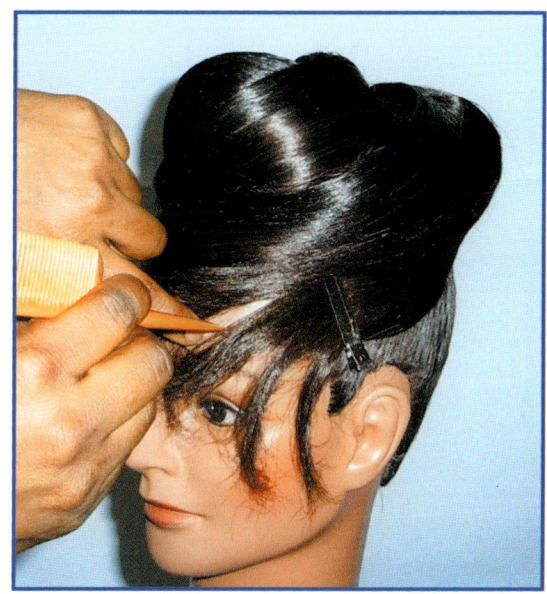

11. Smooth and fan the ends of hair around the face to finish the style.

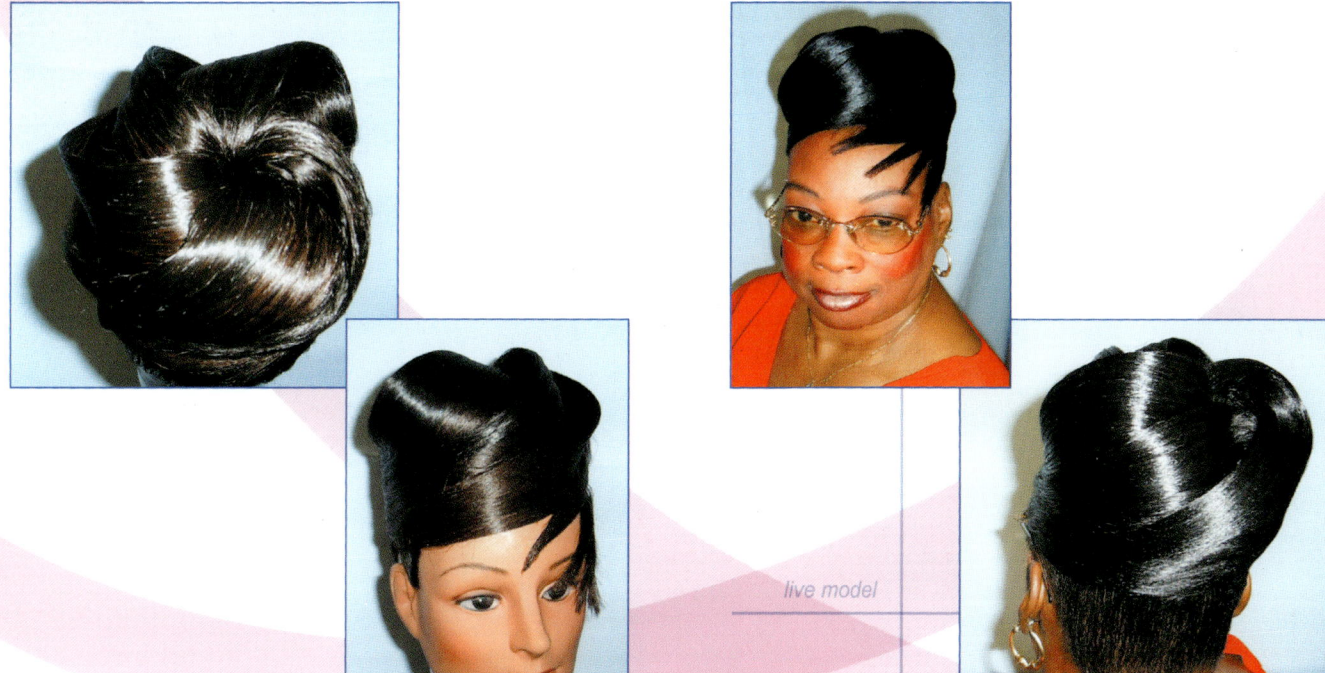

live model

12. Style is complete.

This style is an intricate creation without using any hair pins around the head. A small amount of styling gel smoothed around this design will hold it in place. Dry for 15 minutes. A smooth effect is achieved.

Ponytails

Loops

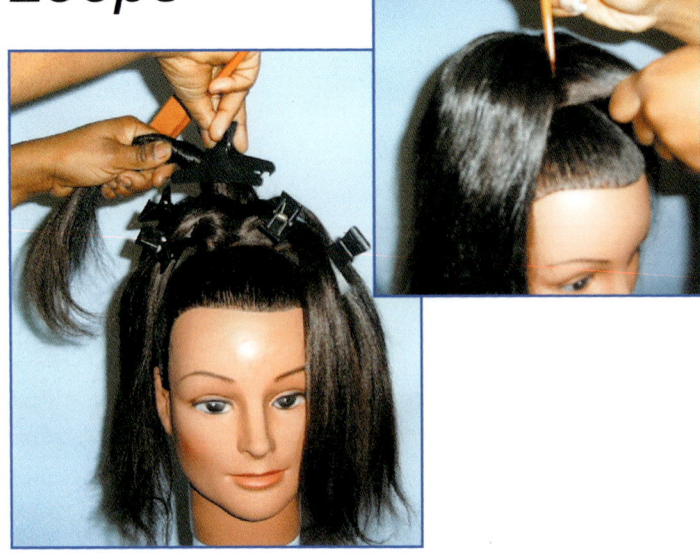

1. Begin by sub sectioning a ponytail into five or six sections.

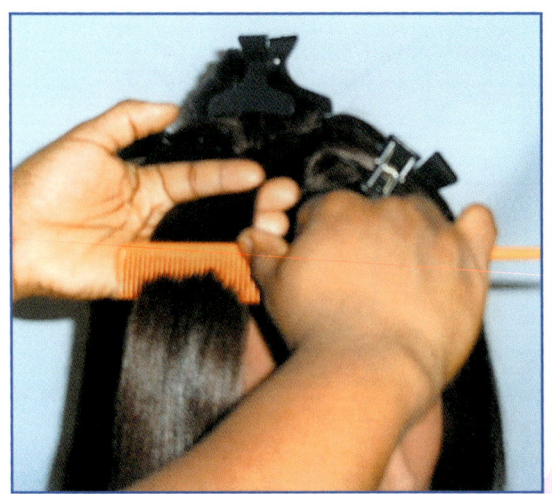

2. Mold a section by directing the hair straight forward.

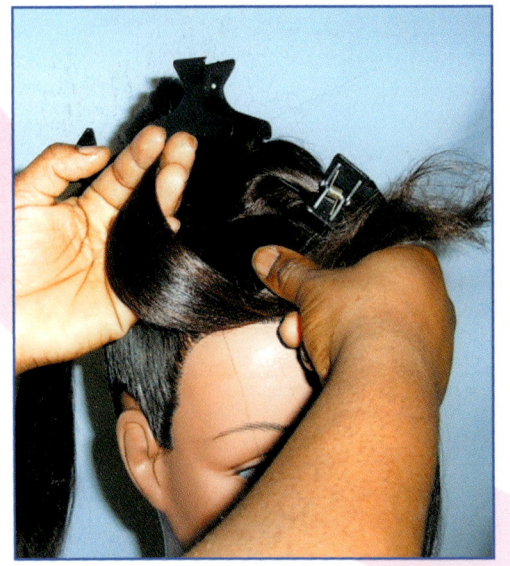

3. Turn Hair in a circular motion.

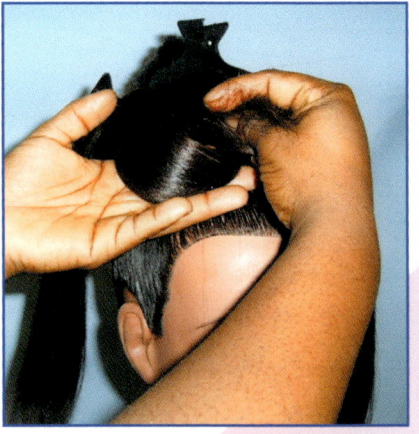

4. Place hair in palm of hand, tuck ends into the circle.

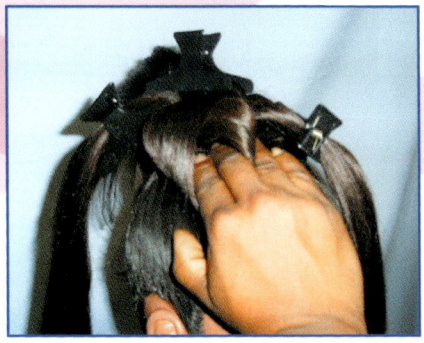

5. Place two fingers in the middle of circle and turn slightly. Place the lopp near the base of the ponytail.

Ponytails

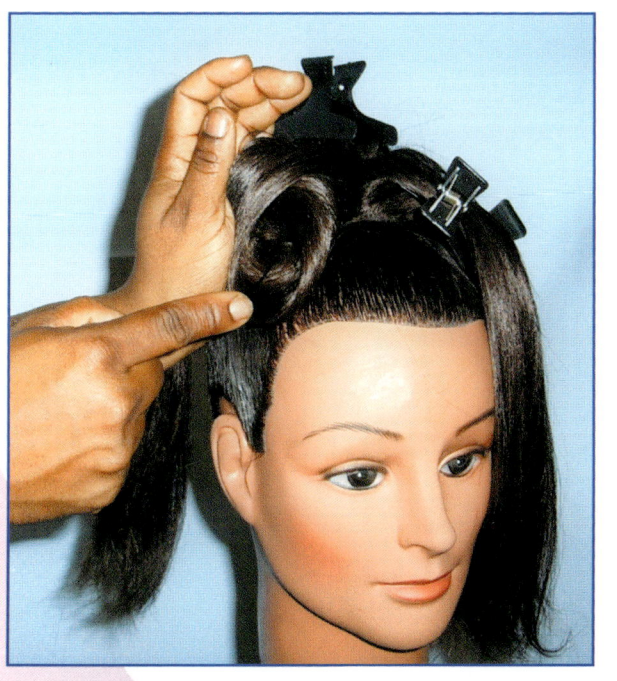

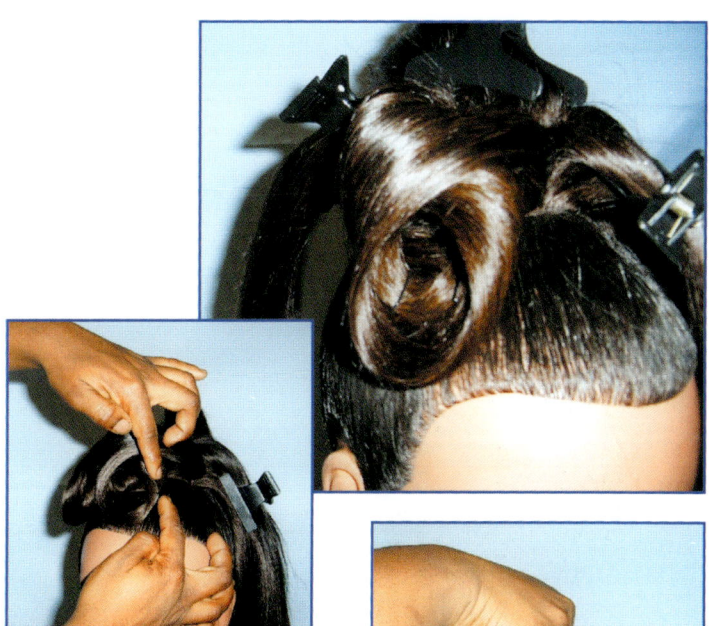

6. Secure with hair pins or bobby pins to the stabilize loop.

7. Continue this technique as you work around the base of the design, making sure each loop is balanced around the head.

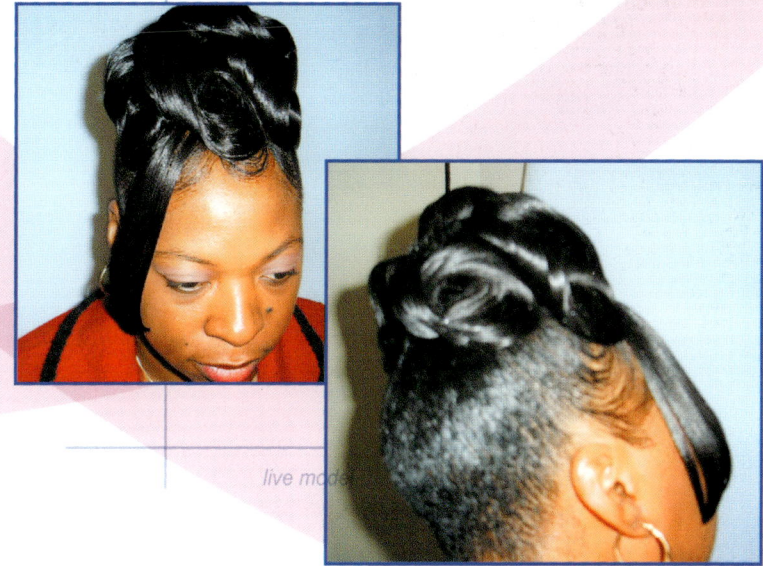

live model

8. This design can be worn for a daytime or evening attraction.

Ponytails

Bun
with pleats

This section is used for pleats at the end of the design.

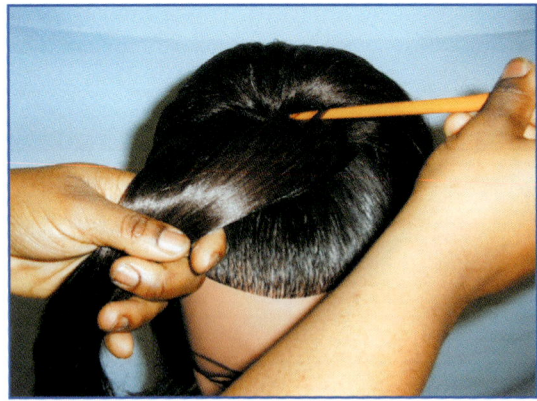
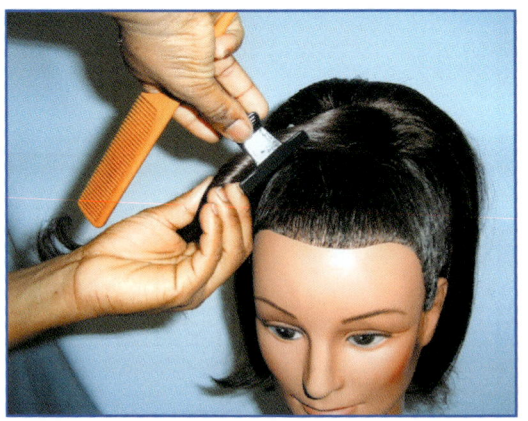

1. Take a horizontal part, starting in front of the ponytail. Two inches of hair should be secured with a jaw clip.

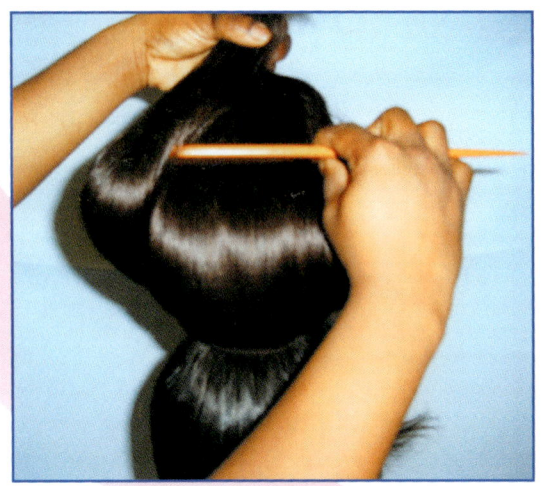
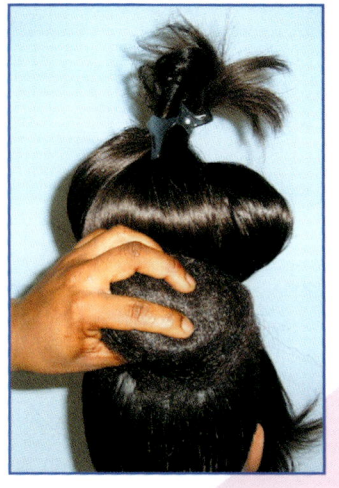

2. Mold remaining ponytail hairs in an upright position.

3. Place hair filler at the base of the ponytail and secure with bobby pins or hair pins.

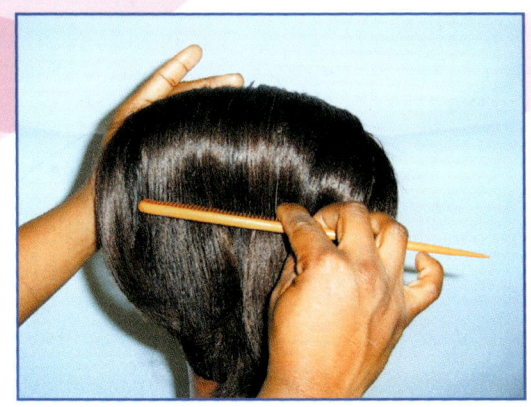

4. Smooth ponytail hair over filler.

Ponytails

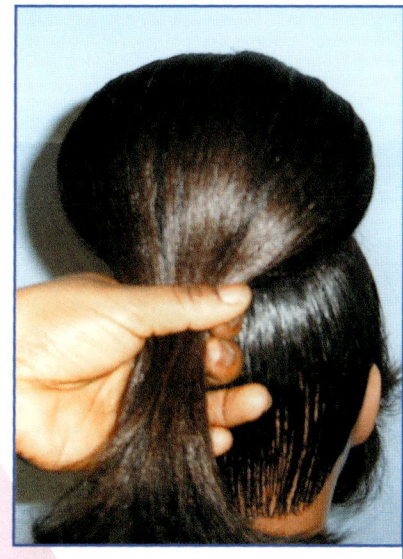
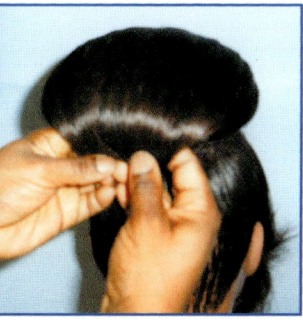

5. Pull hair into a ponytail and tuck hair ends under.

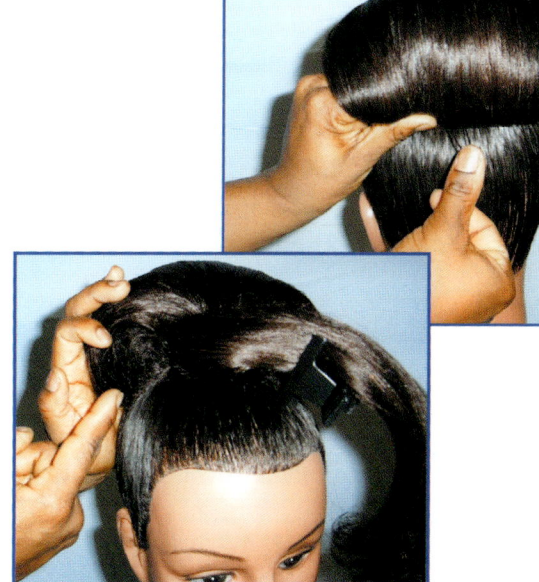

6. Secure with hair pins or bobby pins. Balance bun and secure the open ends on each side.

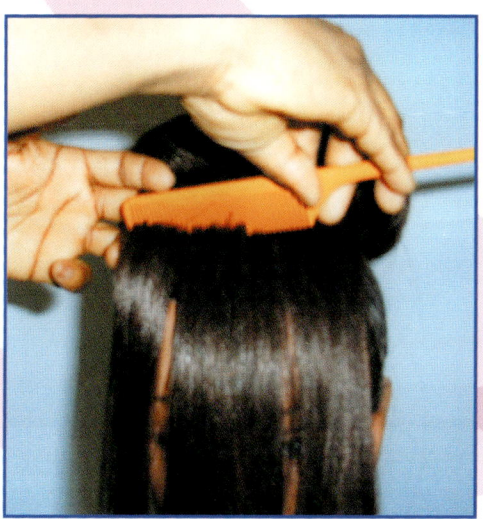

7. The two inch section secured at the beginning of the design is now molded straight forward.

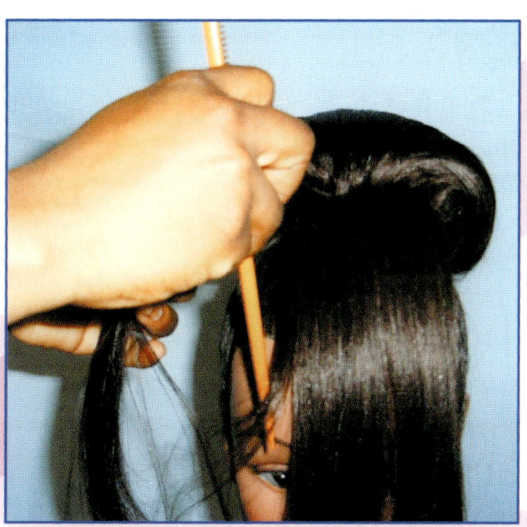

8. Starting from the left side of the head, take a small rectangle for pleats.

Ponytails

Bun
with pleats ...continued

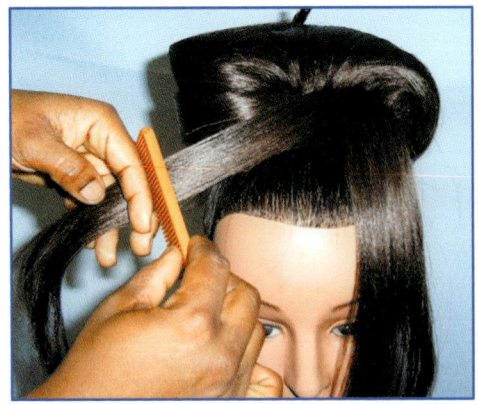

9. A curling iron and holding spray could be used at this time for a more stabilized pleat. Mold hair straight forward.

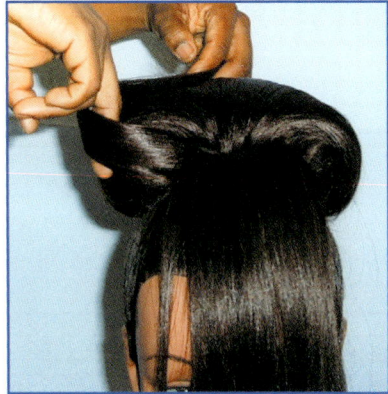

10. Place pleats around the bun and secure ends to bun with a roller clip.

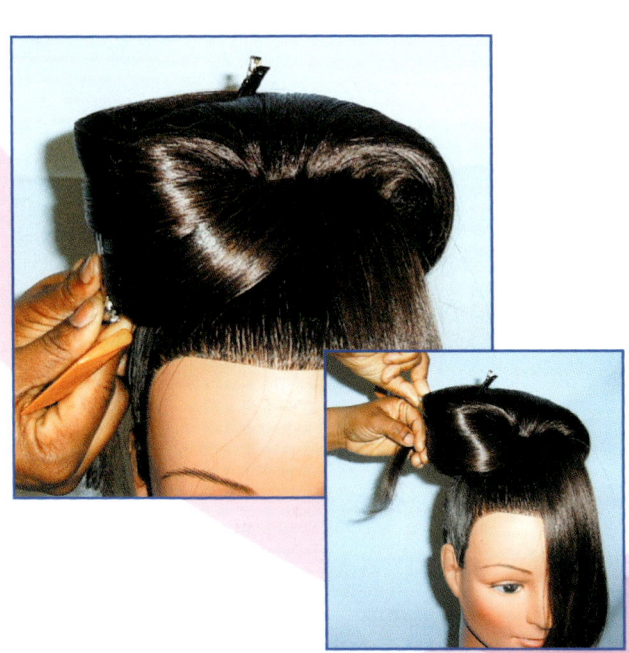

11. Continue to place pleats around the right side of the head, securing hair ends to bun with roller clips.

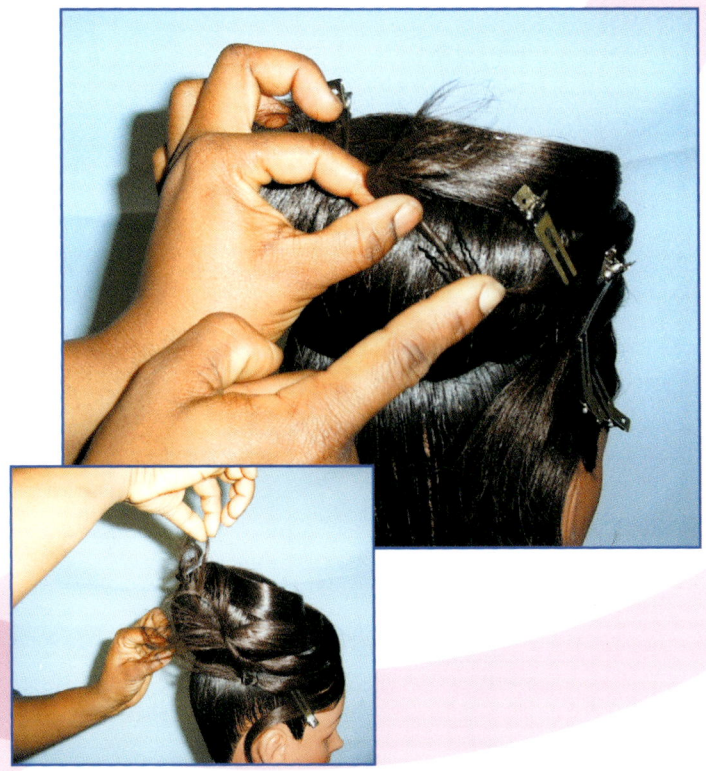

12. Clips are removed and hair pins are used in their place to secure hair ends to the bun. Twist ends of hair and separate strands of hair with your fingers.

Ponytails

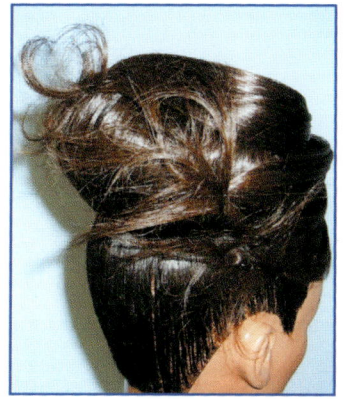 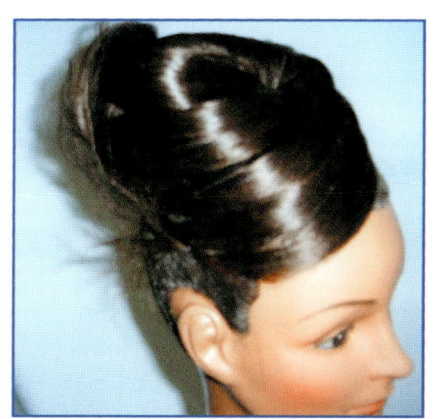 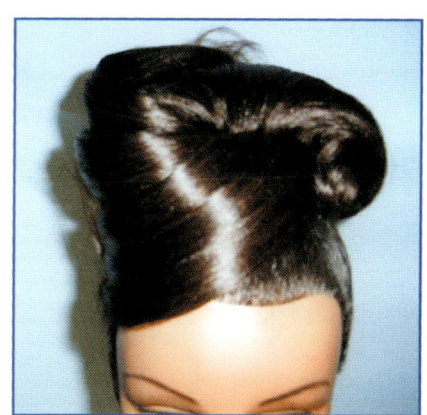

13. An artistically finished design is polished.

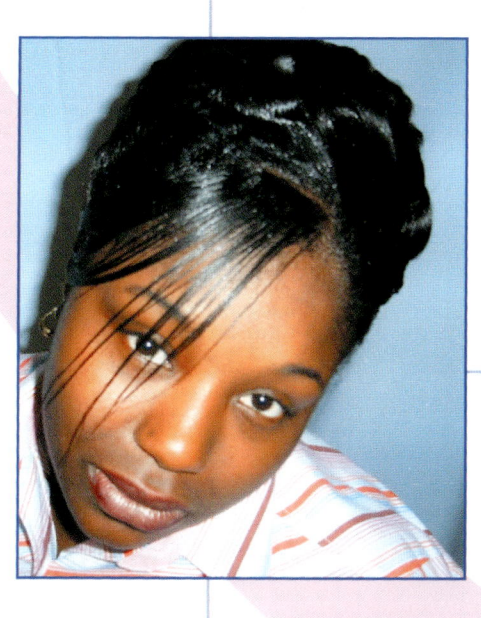

live model

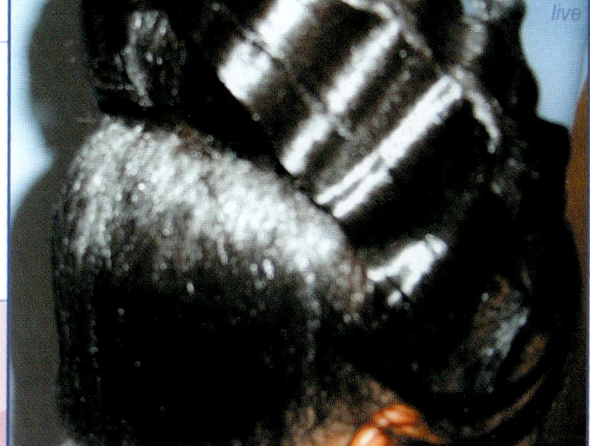

live model

This classical bun design is styled with pleats that are crimped and placed around bun.

Ponytails

Barrel Curl
with pin curl

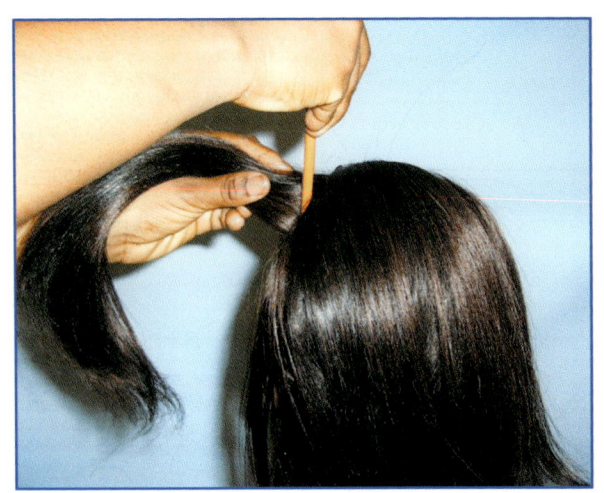
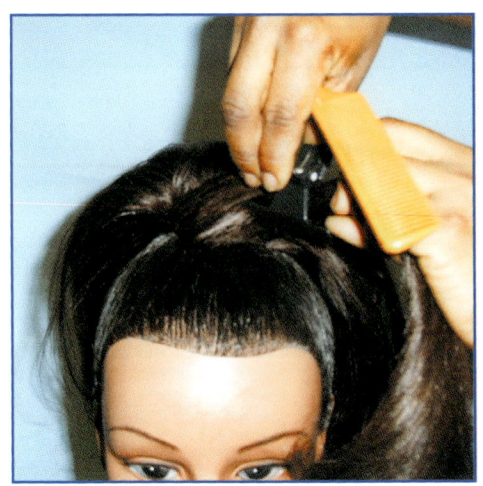

1. Ponytail is carved out in a four inch sub-section in front and secured with a jaw clip. This section will be used later in the illustration for pin curls.

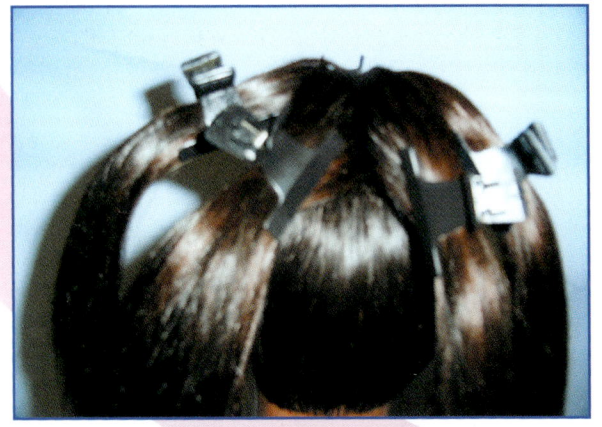
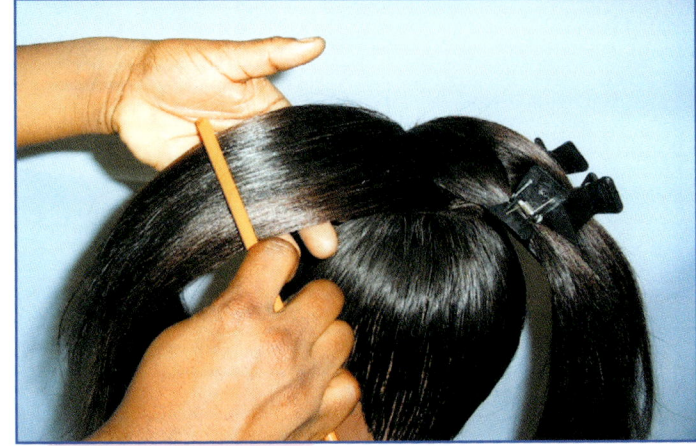

2. The remaining back section is then divided into four sections. Secure with jaw clips. These sections will be used for the barrel curls.

3. Sort from the left by taking a section and smooth out the hair.

4. Hair ends are then placed in the middle. Turn the subsection in an upright position and roll near the base of the ponytail.

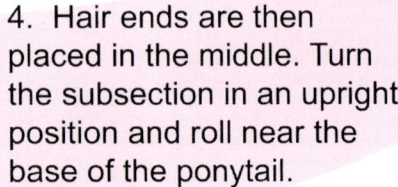
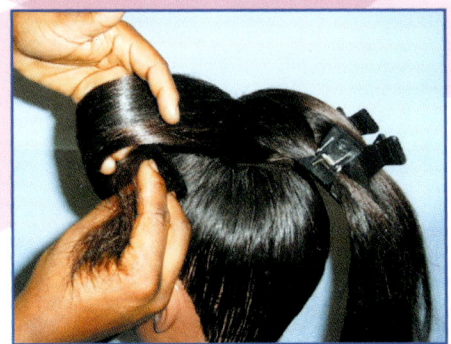
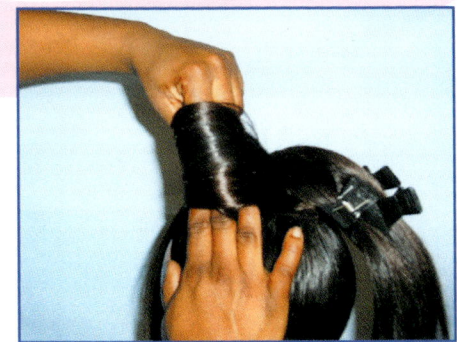

Ponytails

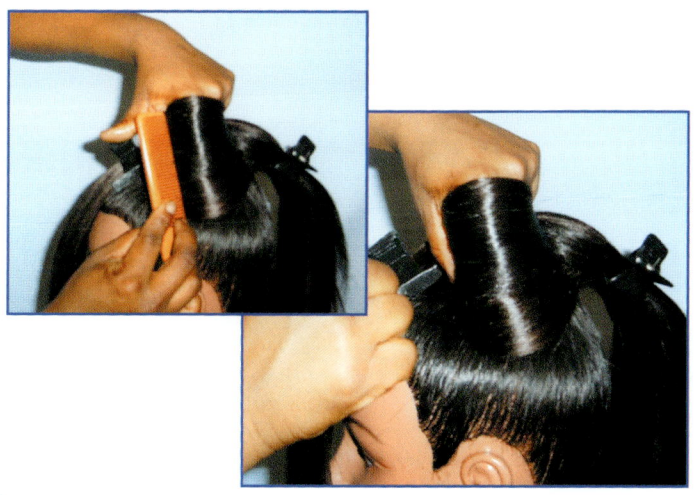

5. Smooth with comb and secure with hair pins at the base of the barrel curl.

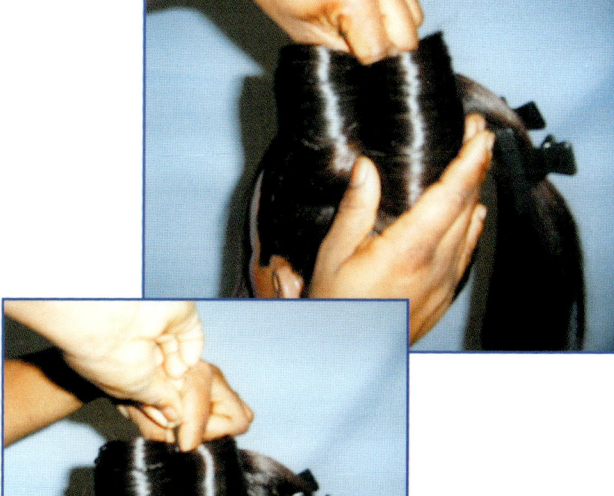

6. Continue the same technique with the remaining subsection and pinch the two together. Place a bobby pin to hold barrel in place.

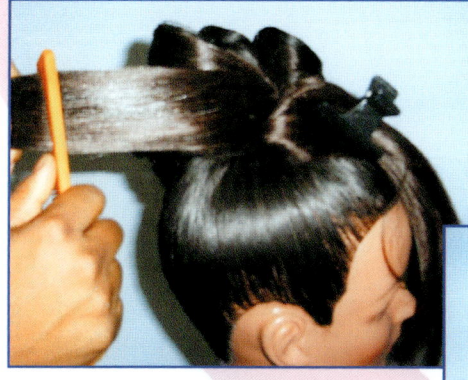

7. The last barrel is smoothed and balanced.

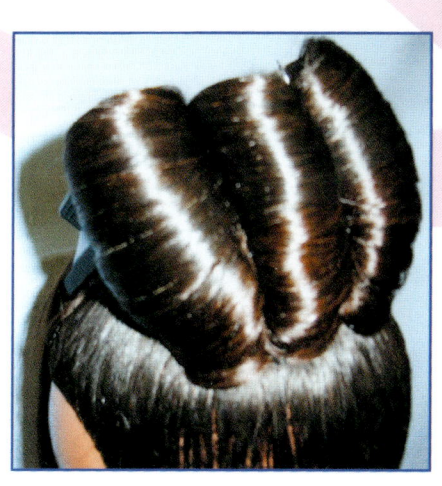

8. Securing hair pins at the base will give a steady hold to this design.

Ponytails

Barrel Curl
with pin curl   ...continued

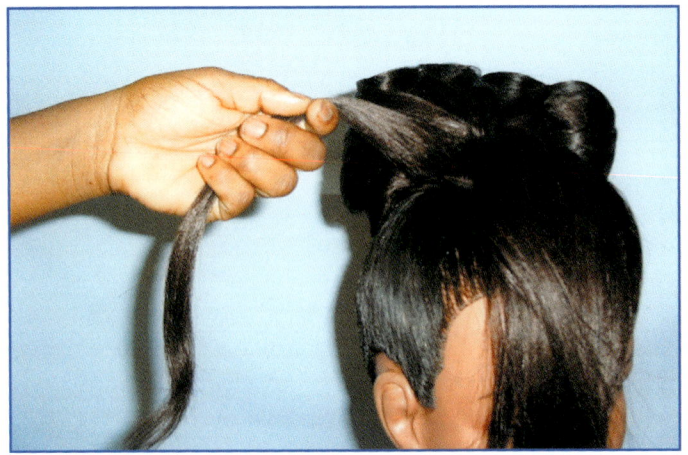

9. The four inch subsection in front is used for the pin curls. Begin by taking a small section of hair.

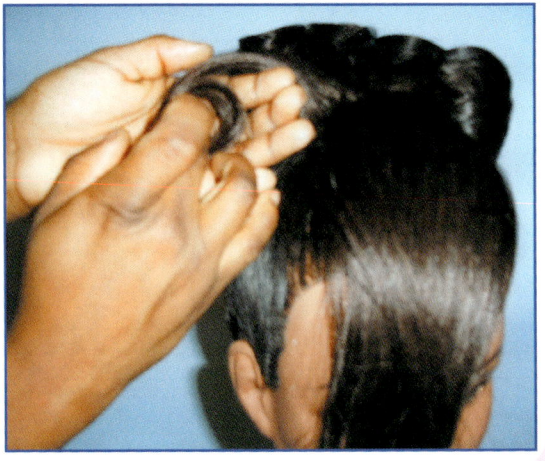

10. Hair ends are rolled and placed in a circle pattern.

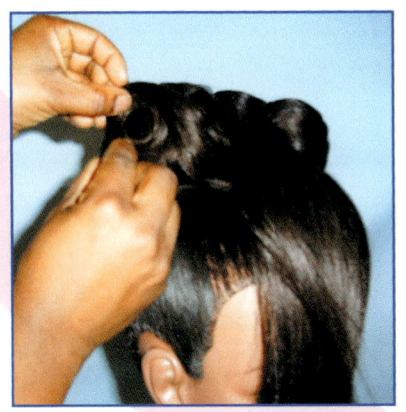

11. Secure pin curl to barrel with hair pins.

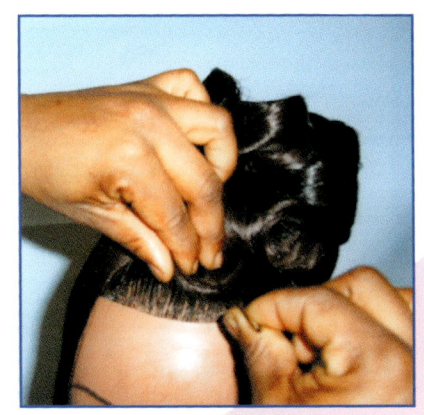

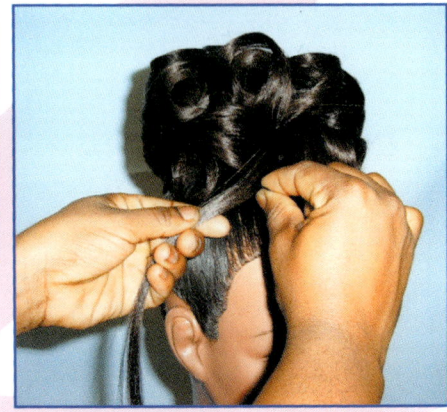

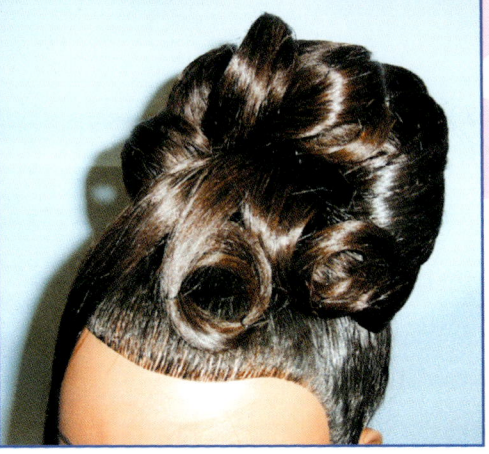

12. Pin curls are set around this design. Individual pieces of hair are used to accent the face. Make sure the style is balanced to finish the design.

Ponytails

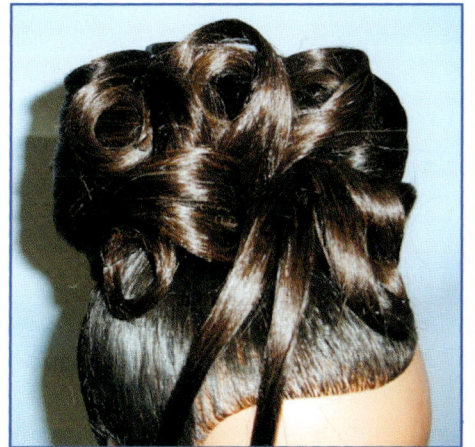
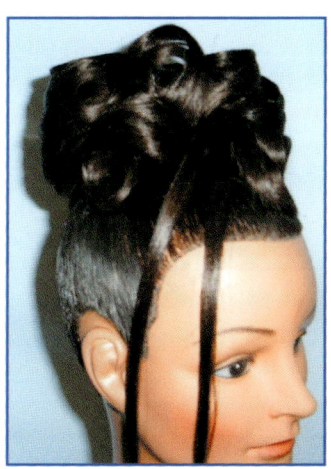
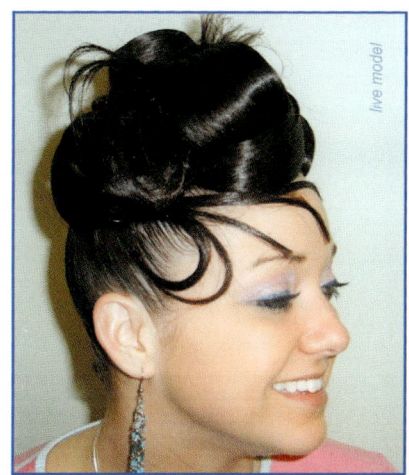

This designer ponytail is set with barrels and pin curls, showing a more conservative look.

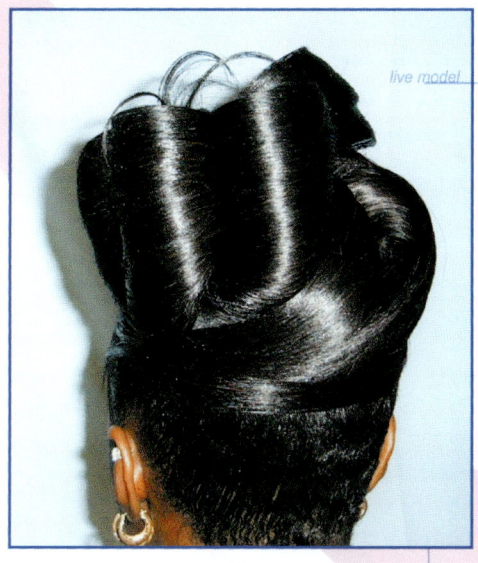

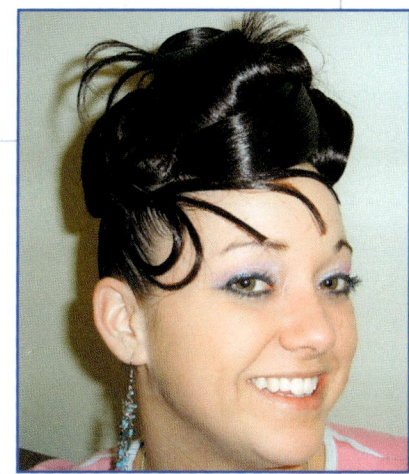

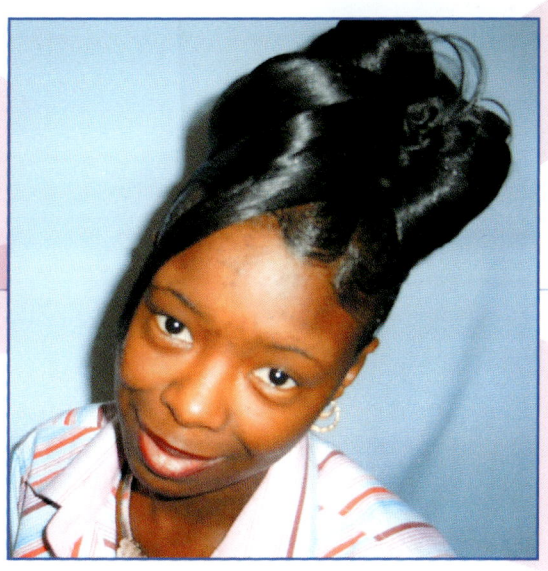

The models above show creative variations.

Ponytails

Stacked Pin Curl

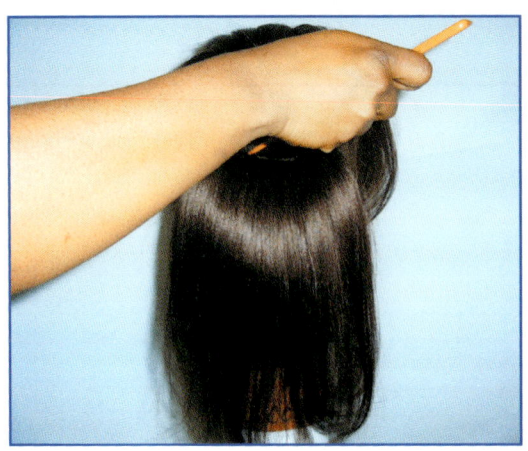

1. Begin the design by scaling out a two inch section in back of the ponytail, securing the remaining ponytail with a jaw clip.

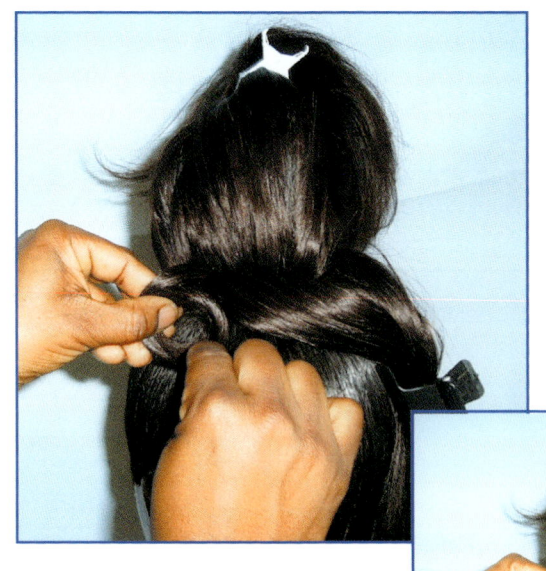

2. From this section, take a small section and secure remaining hair. The small section is then molded in a circular pattern, creating a pin curl. Place pin curl at base of ponytail and secure with hair pin or bobby pins.

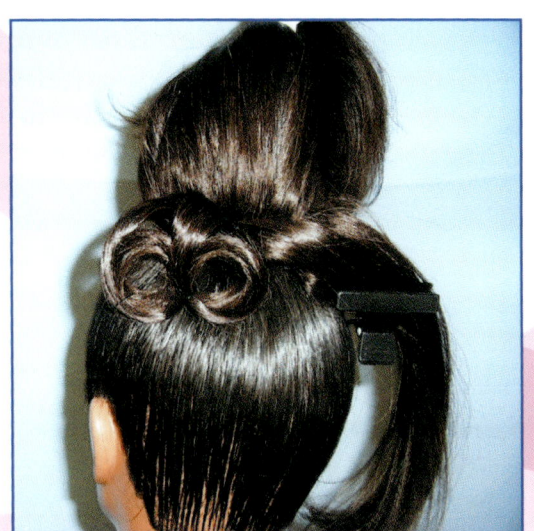

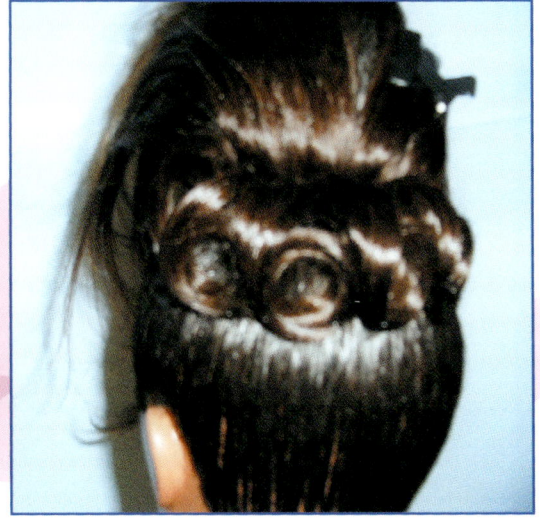

3. Continue this technique, placing the pin curls side by side and securing with bobby pins to the base of the head.

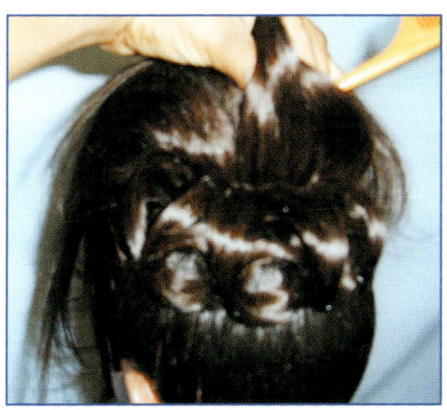 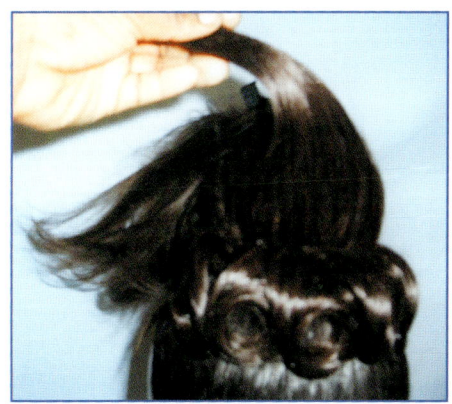

4. To achieve the second row of pin curls, carve out a two inch horizontal section and secure remaining hair with a jaw clip.

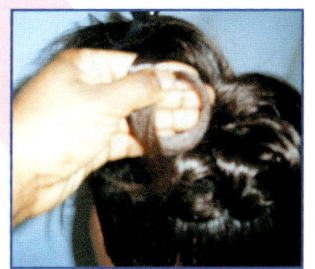 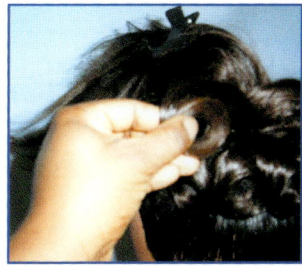

5. Using a small section, continue to design the pin curls.

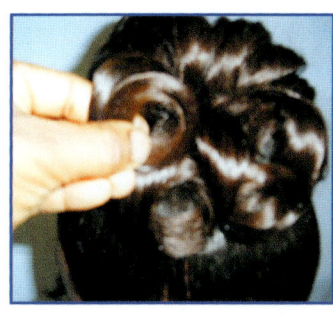

6 Place pin curl on top of previous one. Connect the two together and secure with bobby pins.

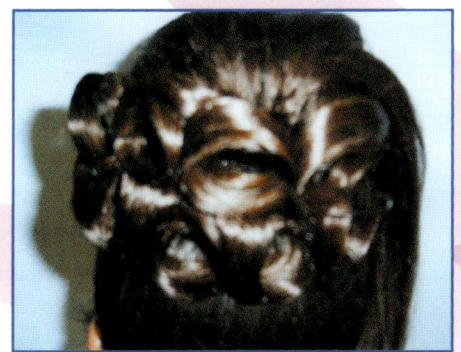

7. Pin curls should stack on top of each other.

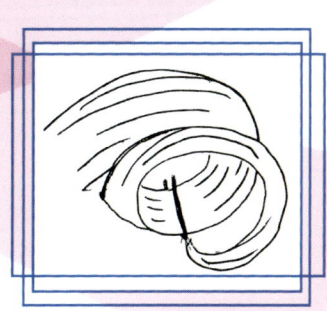

Ponytails

Stacked Pin Curl
...continued

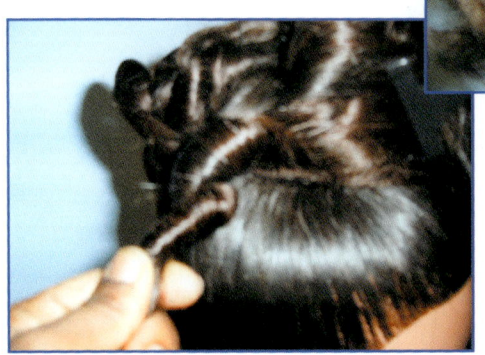

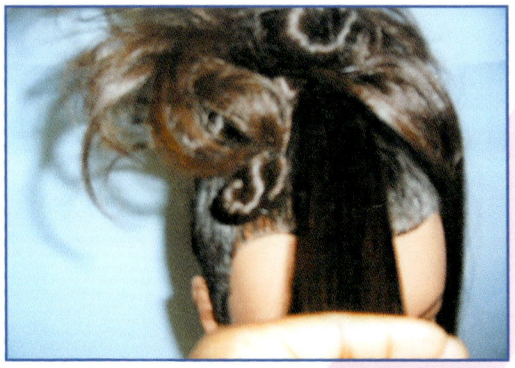

8. A twist design is created in front of the stacked pin curl. Balancing is important at this time. Hair ends are fan-tailed out with your fingers.

9. Bring a small portion to sweep around the face.

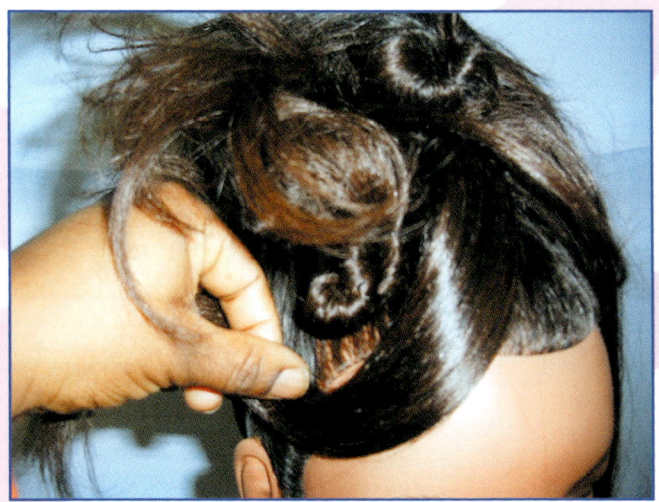

10. Secure with hair pins or bobby pins, continuing to twist the remaining hair strands and create a design with flair.

Ponytails

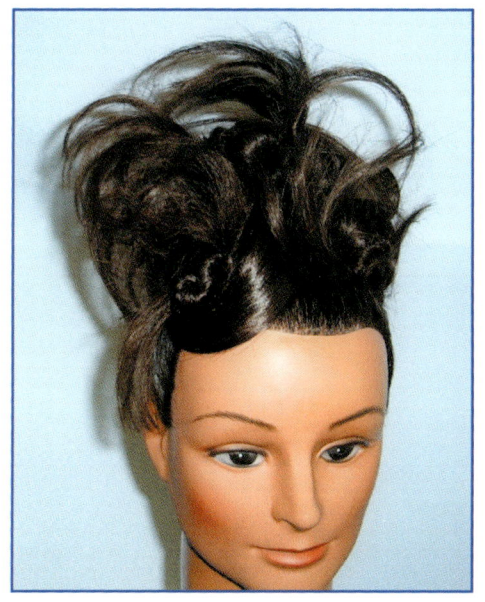
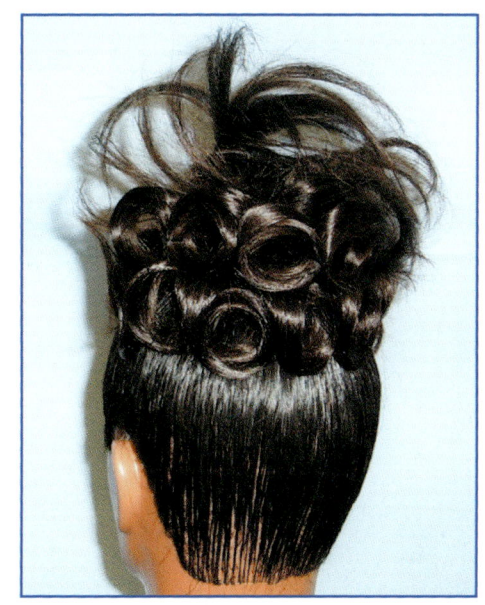

11. Create an artistic design with panache!

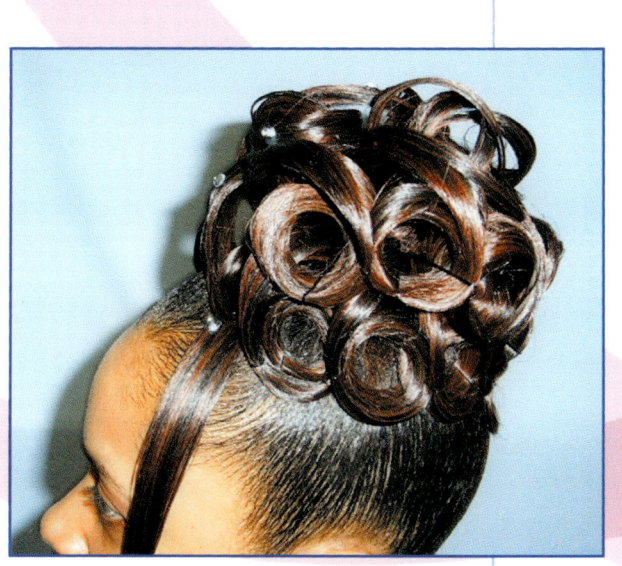
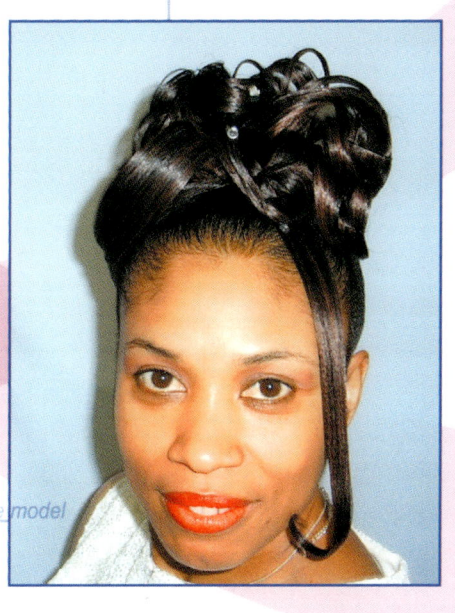

live model

31

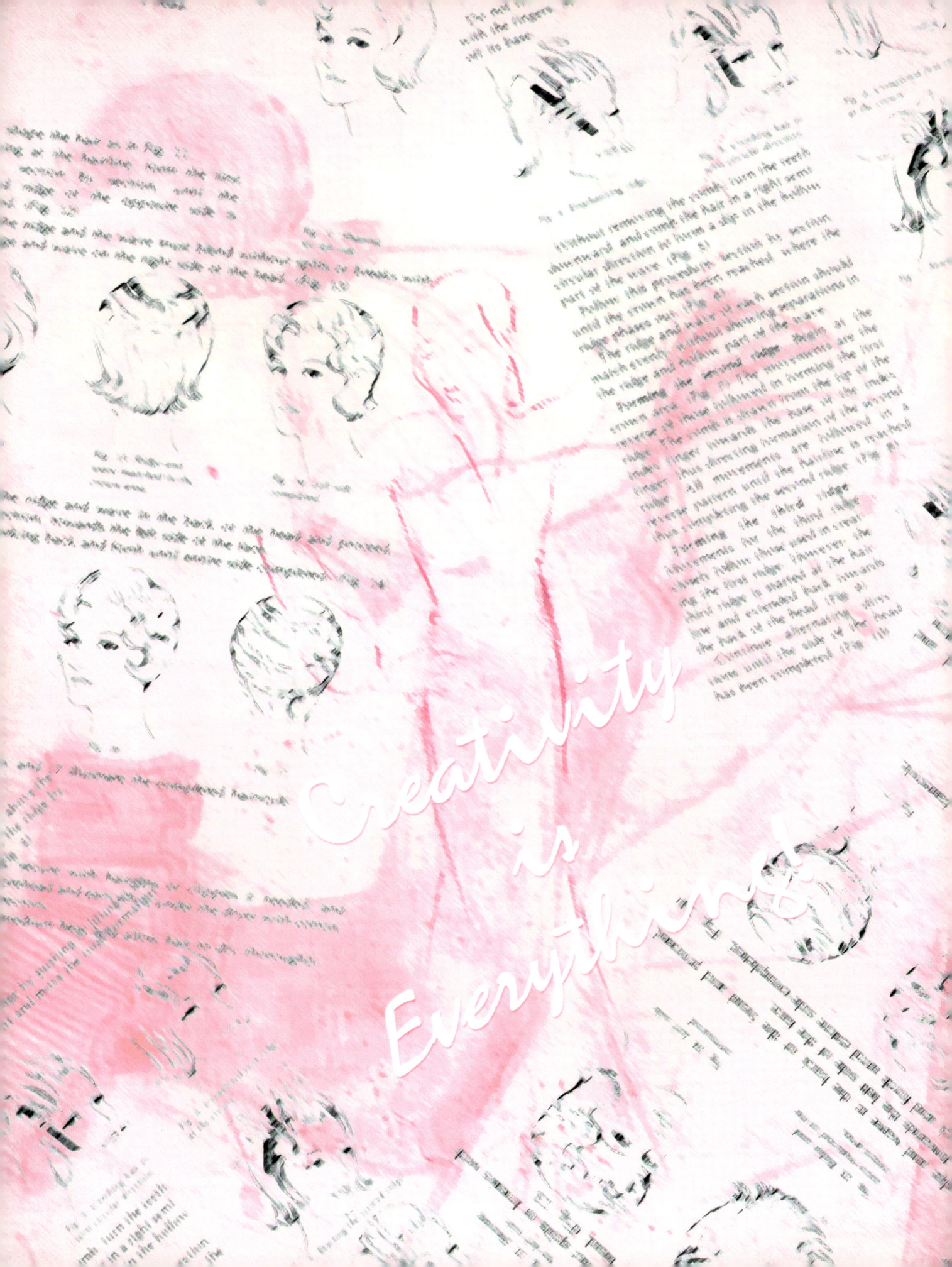

Chapter Three

Twist, Coils & Fingerwaves

3

Fingerwave
with curls

A fingerwave is created by two complete alternating oblongs. This technique can be designed to enhance any style. It also can be done with your fingers or the two comb method.

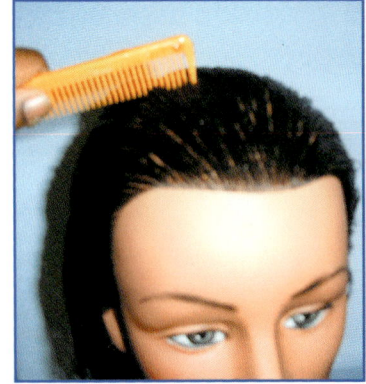

1. Begin by placing gel on wet hair.

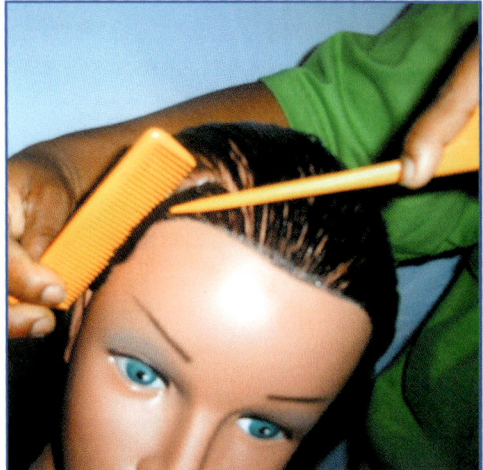
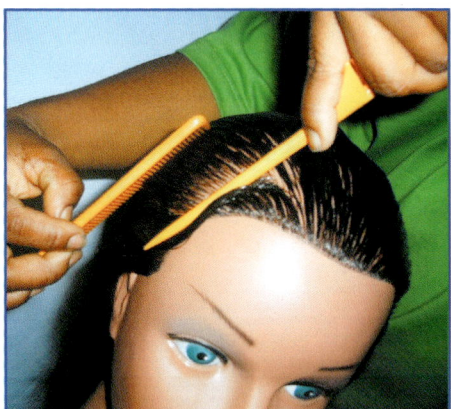

2. Mold hair in the direction you wish to start. Place tail comb at hairline. The comb is then used to create the first ridge.

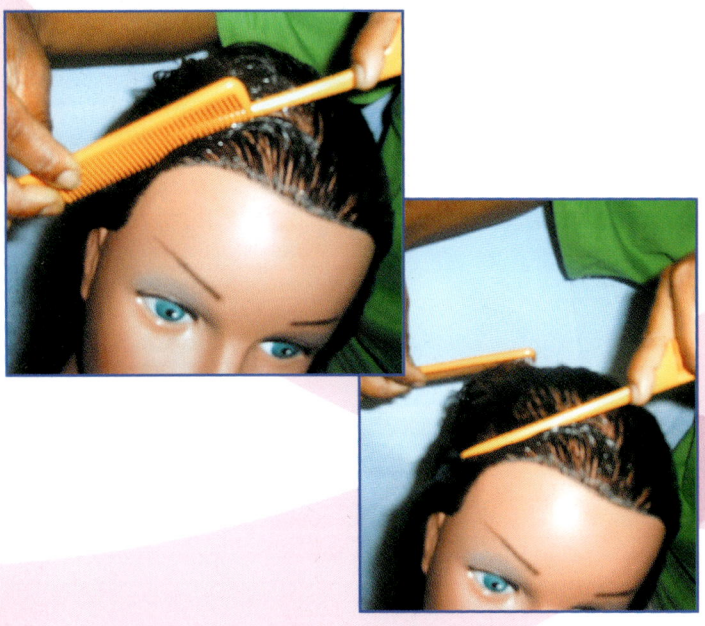

3. Hold the tale comb firmley against the ridge. Use the opposite comb to comb tangles out of the hair.

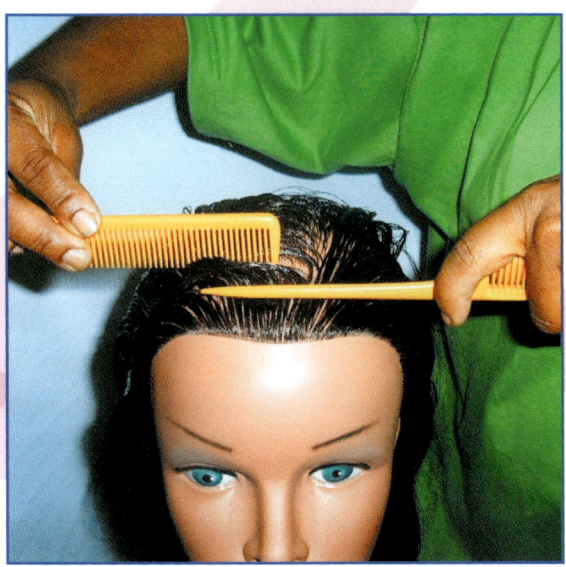

4. Continue this technique across the front.

Twist, Coils & Fingerwaves

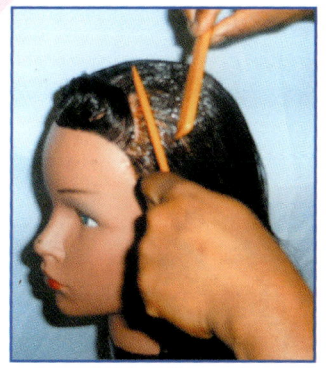 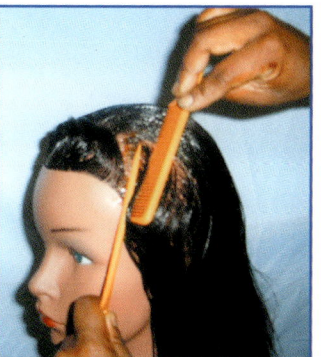 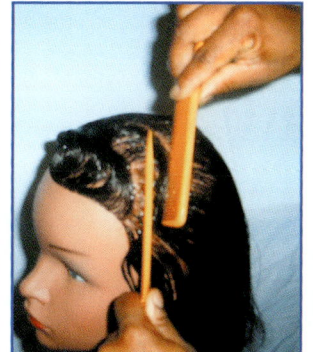 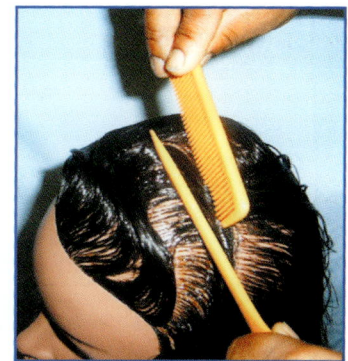

5. This should complete the first ridge.

6. Starting one half inch back behind the previous ridge, mold hair in the direction the hair is going. This should be the open oblong. Continue the same technique, creating a second ridge.

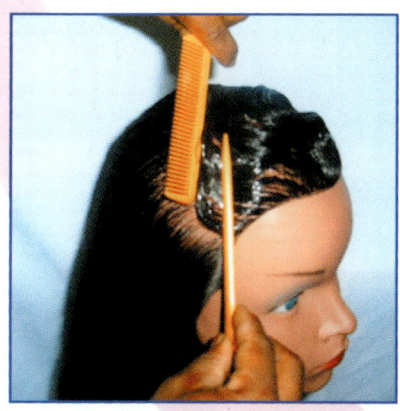 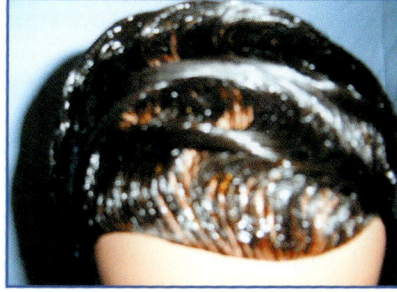 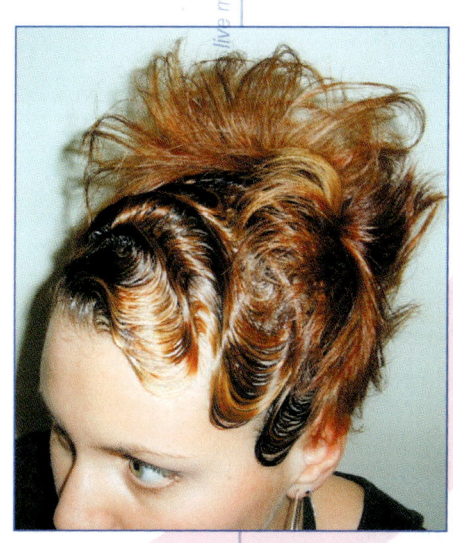

7. The second ridge should be closed at the end. This should define an alternating oblong pattern.

8. Continue to mold hair in the next direction, using the same technique to make the third ridge. Dry hair and style as desired.

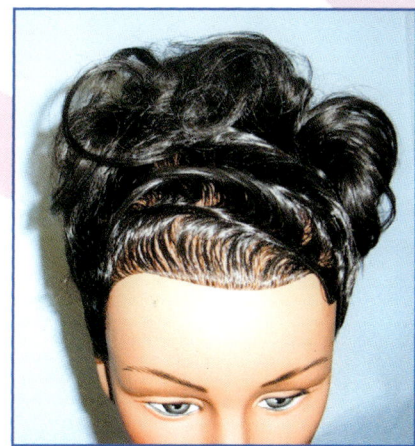 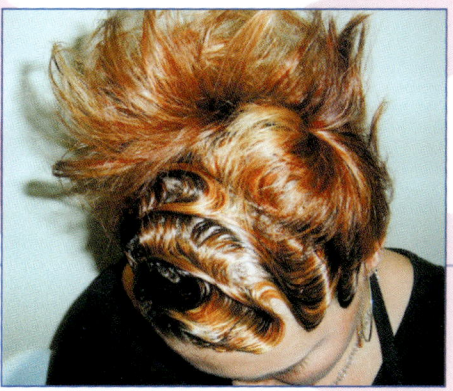

9. Remaining hair is curled and styled with elegance.

This style can be curled, set on rollers, or styled with a french roll, if desired.

35

Twist, Coils & Fingerwaves

Flat Twist
with water falls

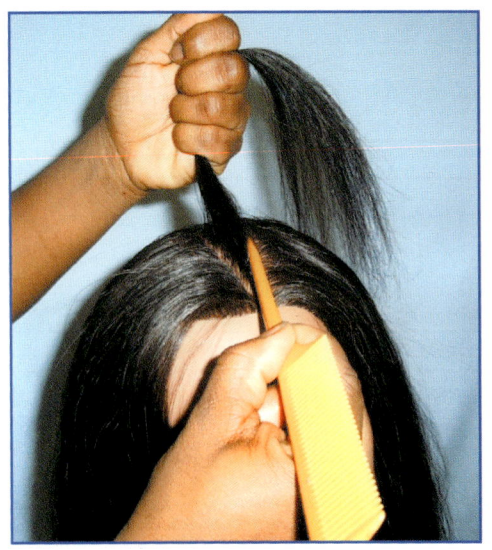

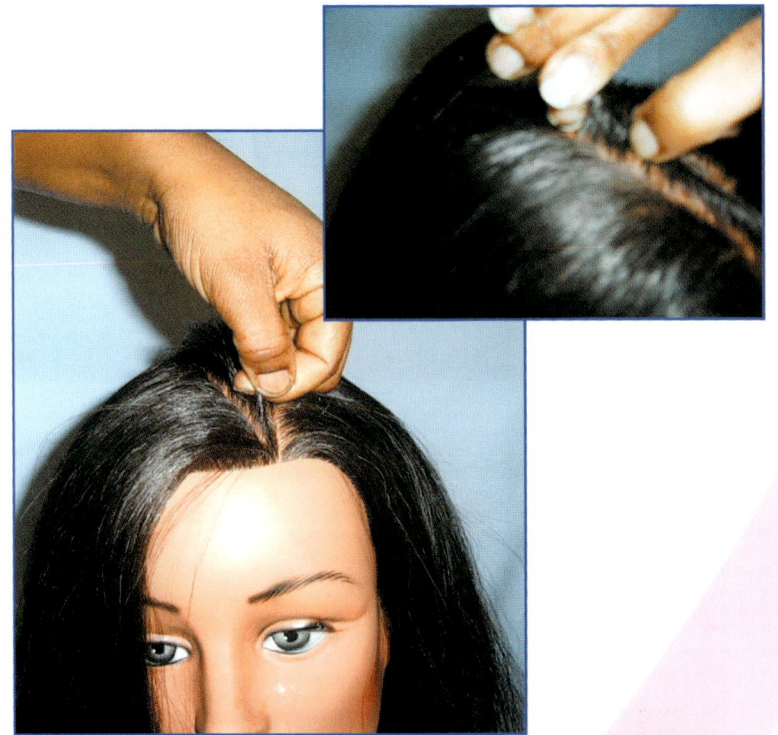

1. Start by parting out a thin vertical section.

2. Begin to twist hair at the beginning of the part. Continue to twist and pinch hair together, creating a flat twist as you work back towards the crown area.

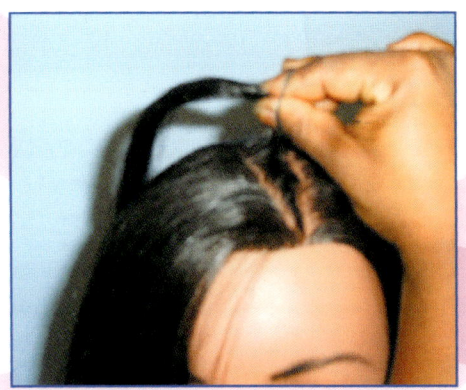
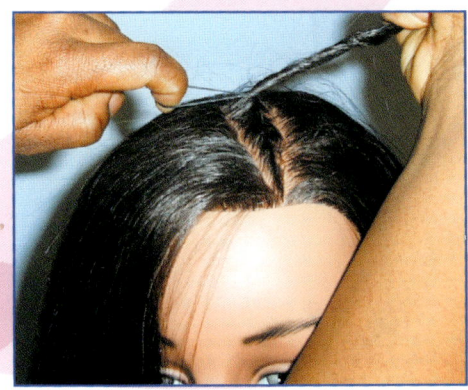

3. Coil hair at the end of the twist and place a rubber band to hold in place.

Twist, Coils & Fingerwaves

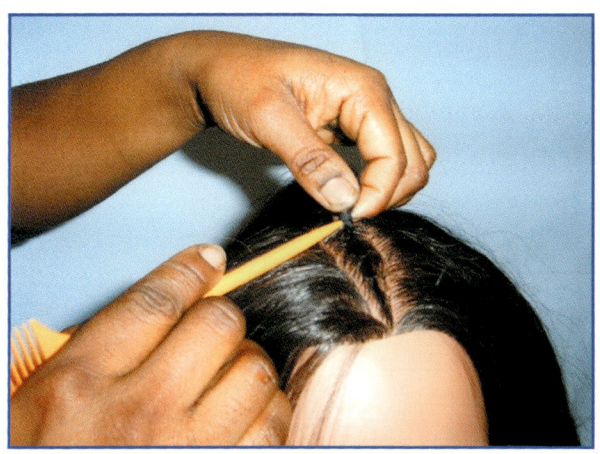

4. Make sure the rubber band is secure in place. The twist should not unravel, giving a tight hold.

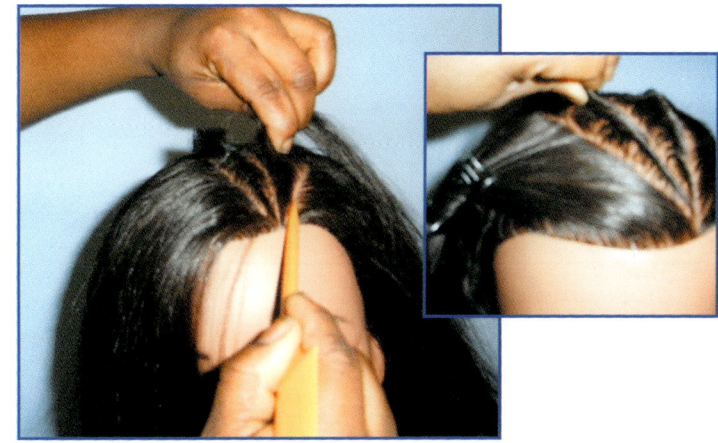

5. Continue to part from the point of the previous twist. The flat twist should come from one point of origin.

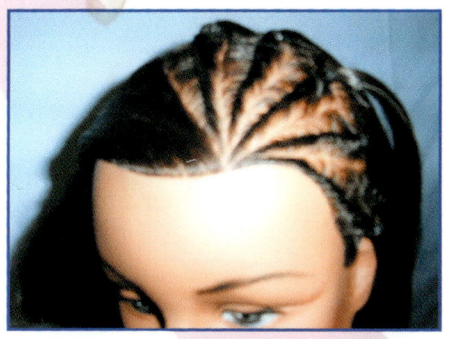

6. The remaining twist should come from the same point, creating a half-circle.

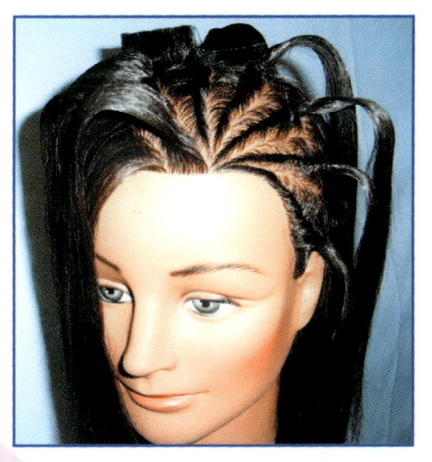

7. The flat twist is then finished out with waterfalls. Providing you with a flamboyant appearance.

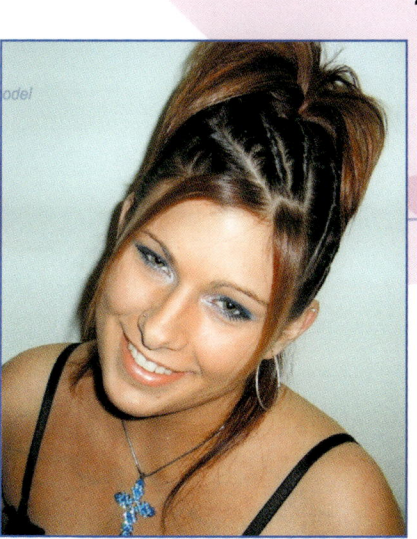

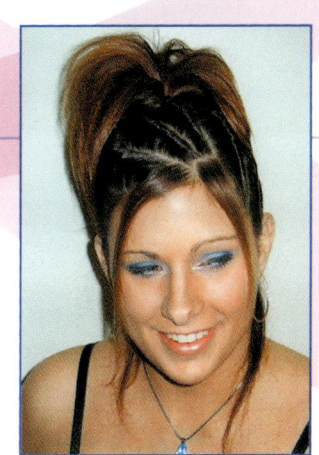

Twist, Coils & Fingerwaves

Flat Twist
with weave

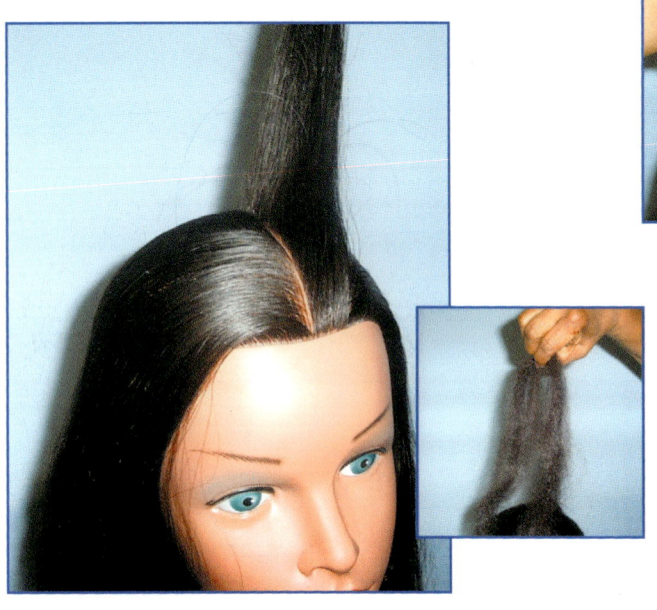

1. Begin by parting out a thin vertical section of hair. A small amount of hair filler is used for this design.

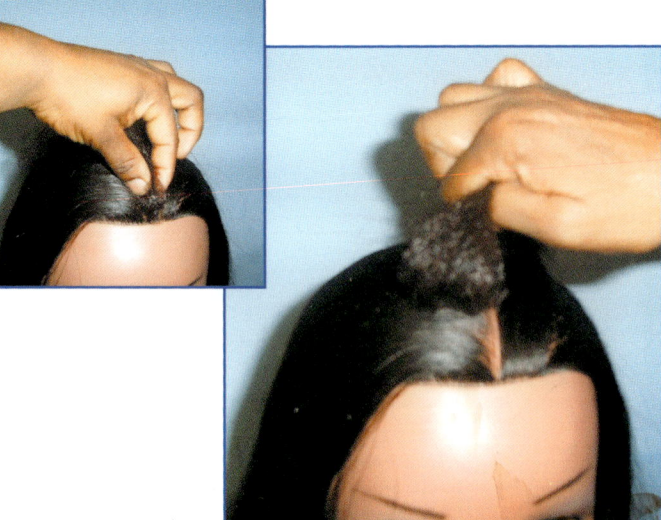

2. Place filler along the part.

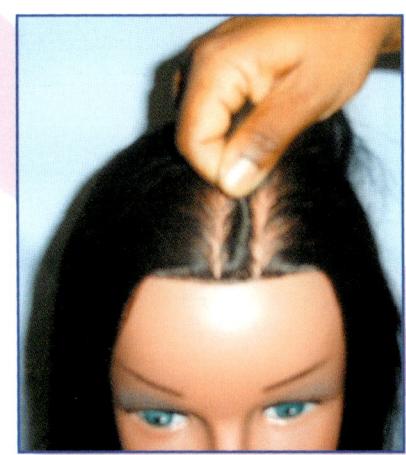

3. Start twisting natural hair over filler.

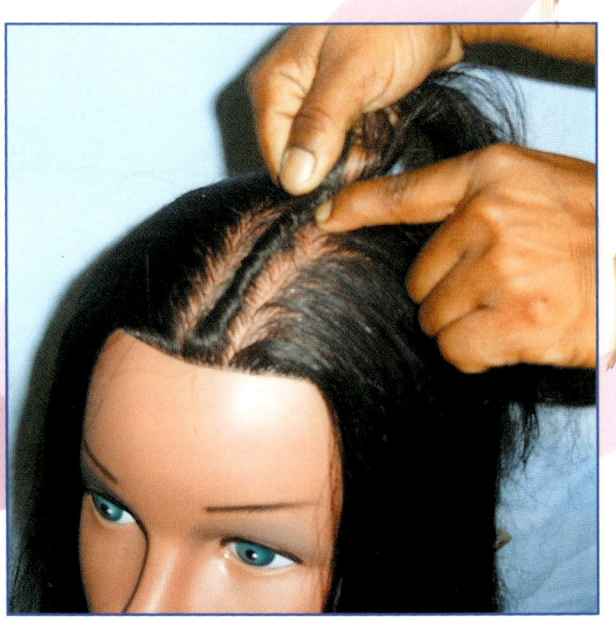

4. Continue to twist natural hair over filler.

Twist, Coils & Fingerwaves

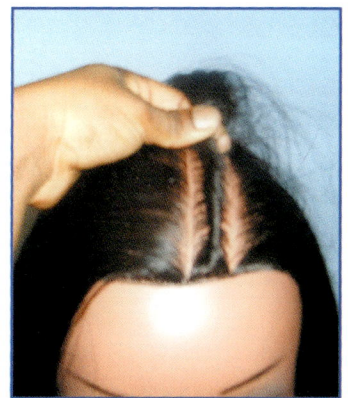 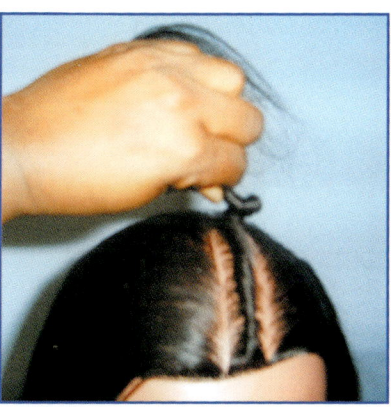

5. The filler is used to create a firm flat twist. Coil ends tightly.

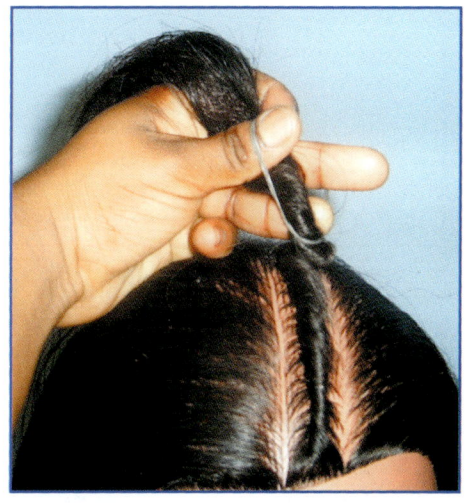

6. Place a rubber band at the base of the flat twist.

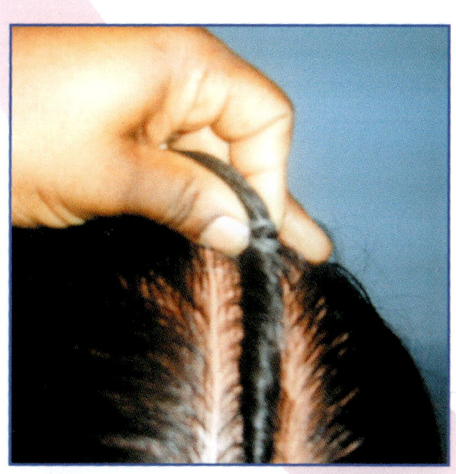

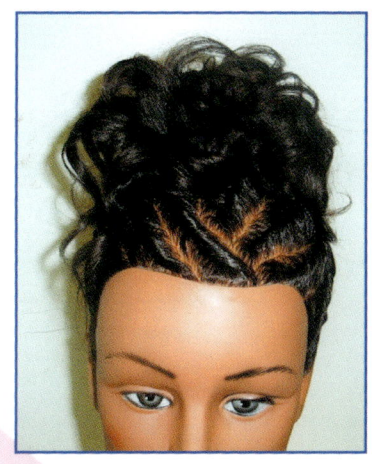

8. This design is a fashion statement. Adding filler to the hair will ensure a steady flat twist on the scalp. This technique is a work of art.

7. This gives a strong hold. A flat twist on the scalp is created.

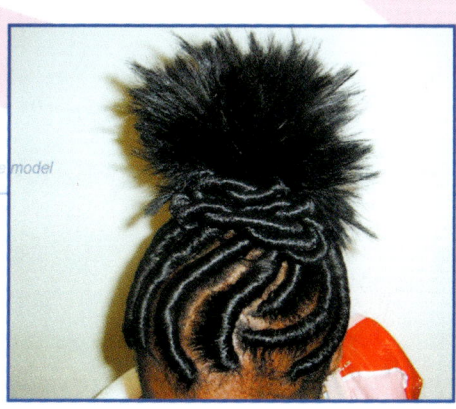 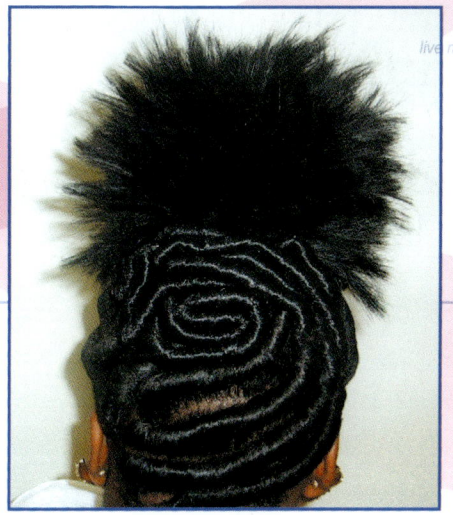

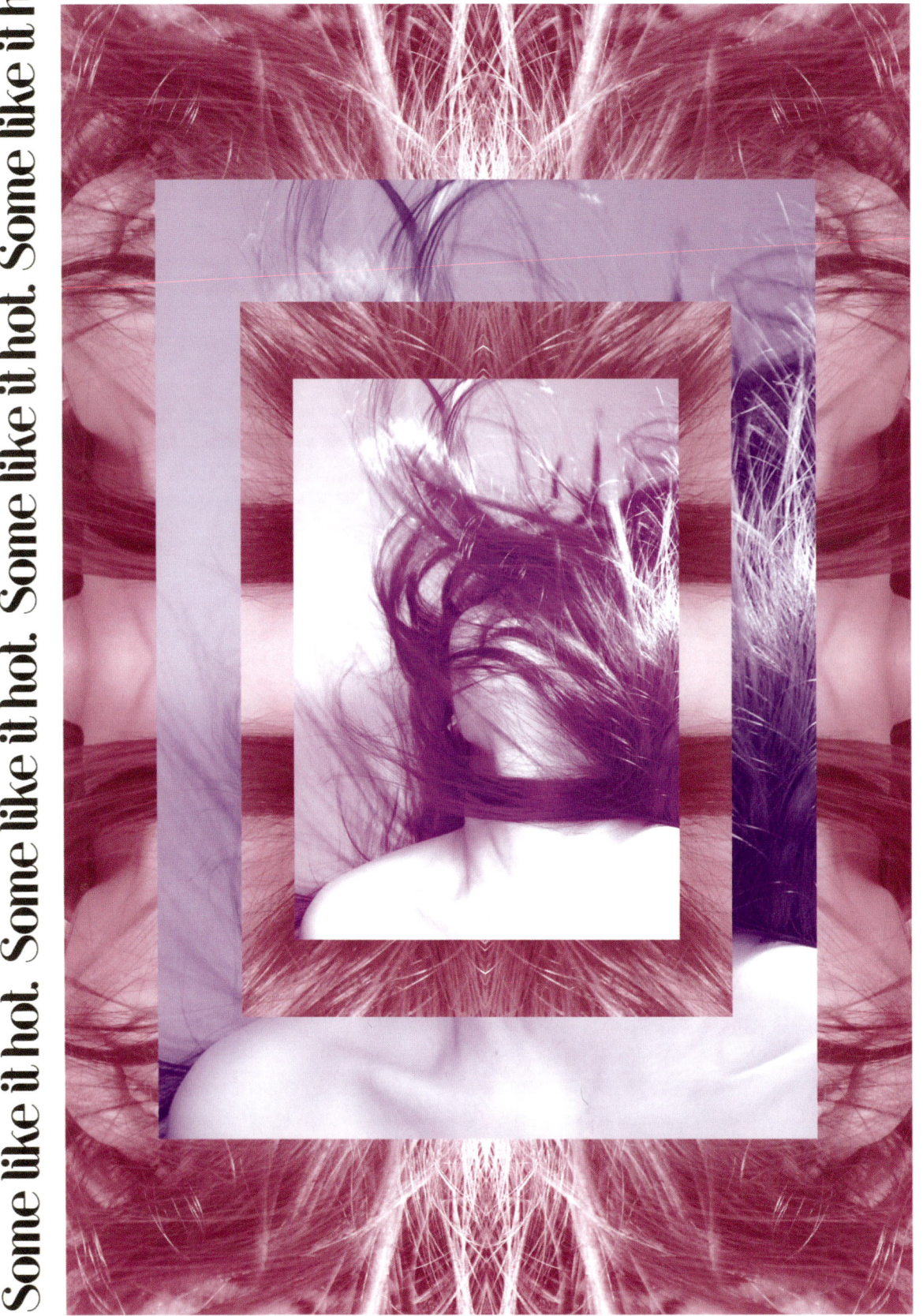

Chapter Four

Thermal Styling

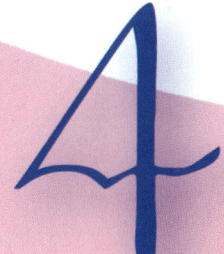

Thermal Styling

Press & Curl

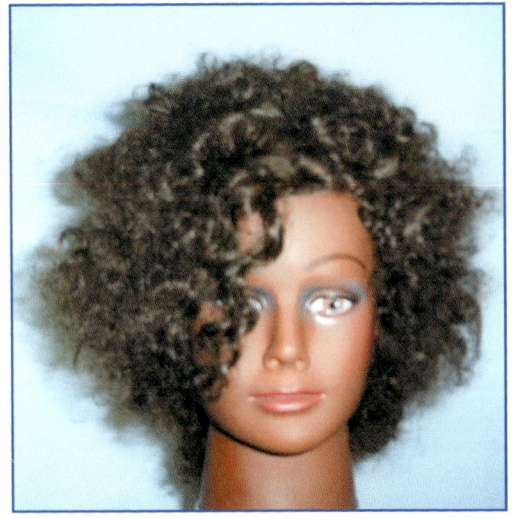

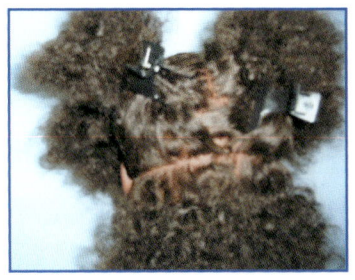

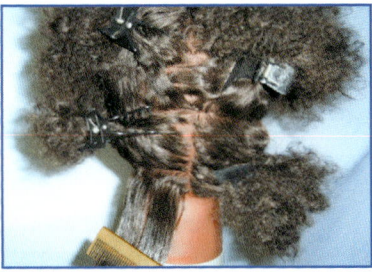

1. Clients with overly curly hair who want to avoid chemicals will usually want a press & curl. This technique is designed to straighten the natural curl.

2. Section the hair into four to five subsections to prepare for the thermal pressing technique.

3. Start pressing hair in the nape area. Use thin sections. Apply pressing oil to hair to protect from the heat.

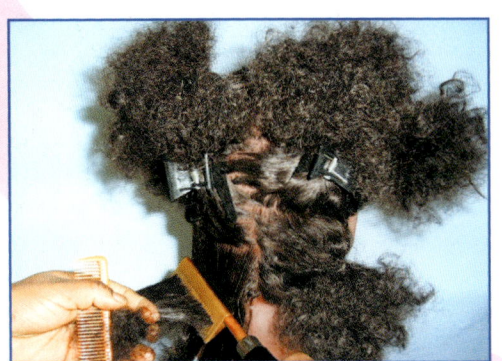

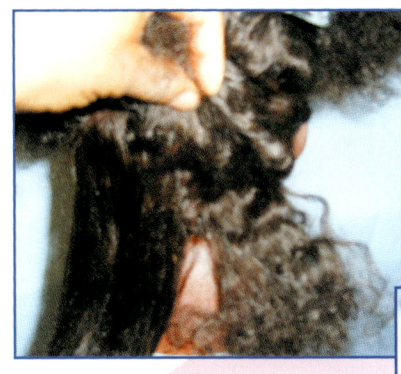

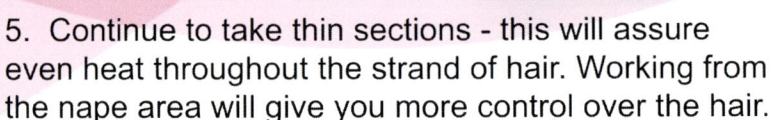

4. Tension is used as you work down the strands of the hair.

5. Continue to take thin sections - this will assure even heat throughout the strand of hair. Working from the nape area will give you more control over the hair.

Thermal Styling

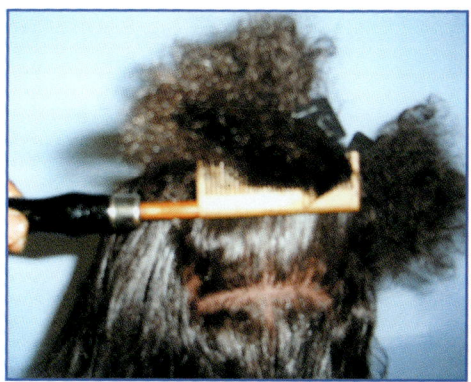

6. Turn the pressing comb and press the hair with the spine as you work up and under from the base to the hair ends.

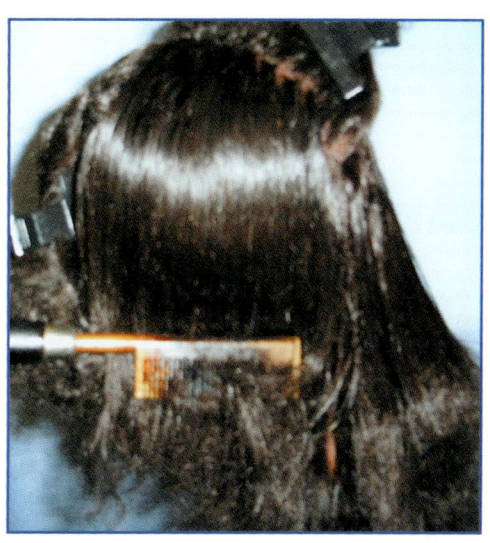

7. Repeat this technique twice for each new subsection.

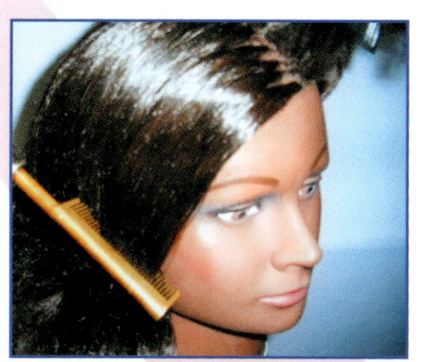

8. Press the hairline last. Once the hair is completely pressed, you may perform a haircut, if desired.

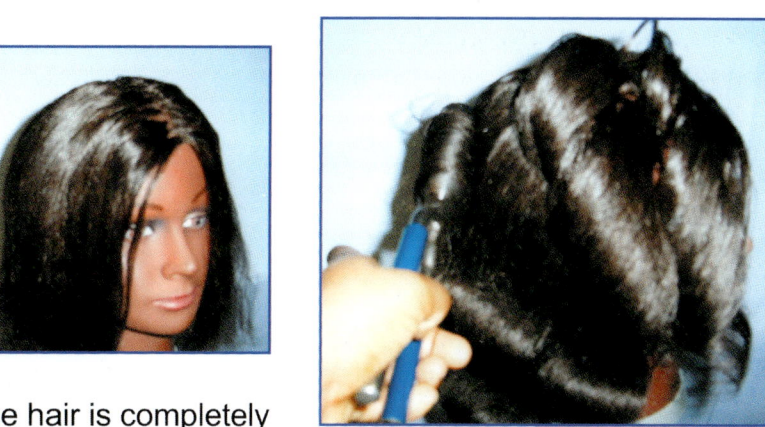

9. Curl with a Marcel curling iron.

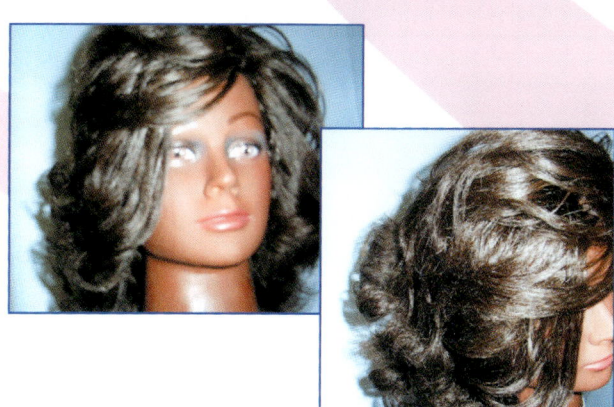

10. Balance and complete the comb out.

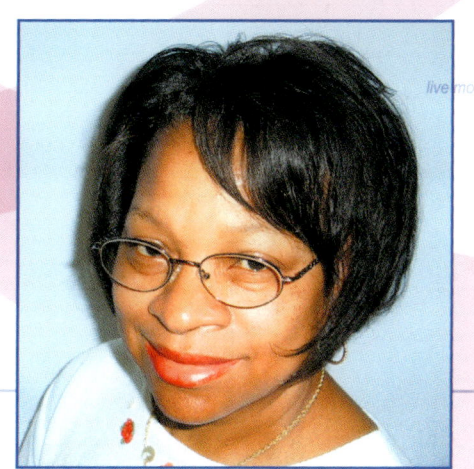

43

Thermal Styling

Marcel Curling Iron

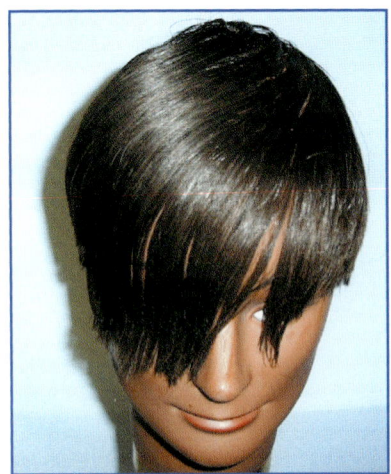
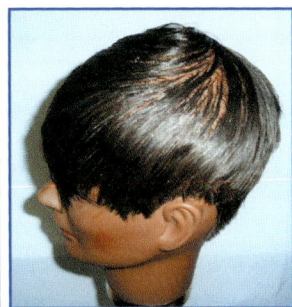
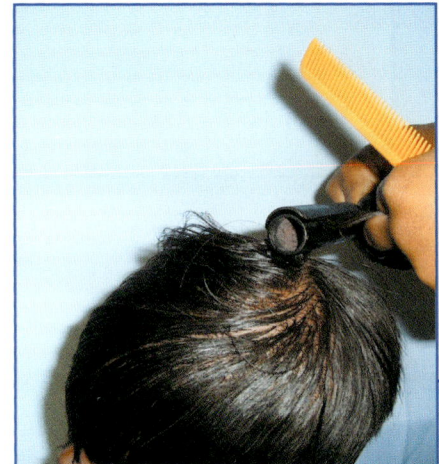

1. Hair is shampooed, molded flat, and dried in the direction you desire to curl.

2. Starting in the crown area. Place the tongs near the base of the head. Rotate the tongs to free the hair as you work up towards the ends of the hair..

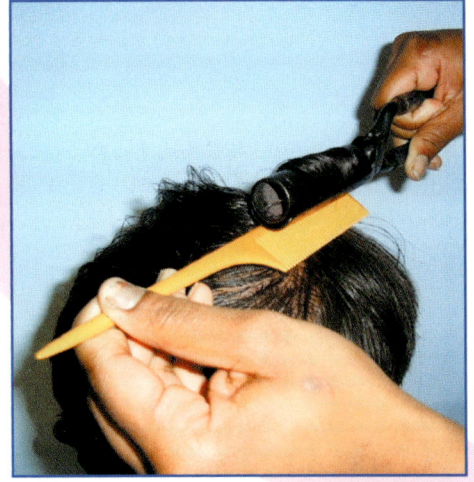
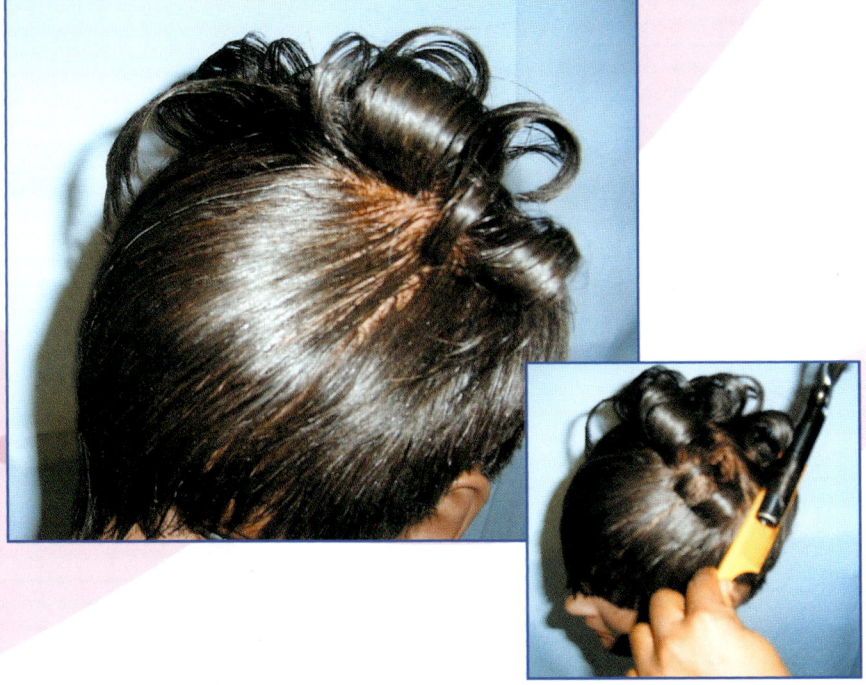

3. The use of a hard rubber comb will protect you from going to close to the scalp.

4. Continue to curl in the direction the hair was molded.

Thermal Styling

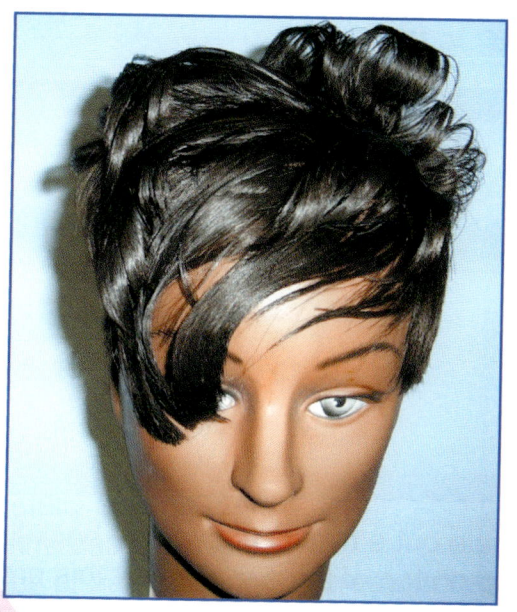

5. Slide curls are used around the face. Let curls cool before you begin to style.

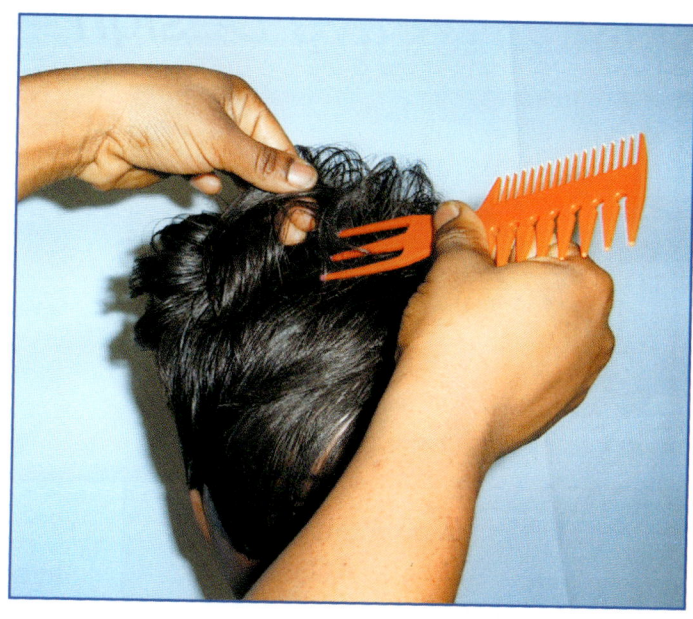

6. Style with a three in one styling comb or your preference.

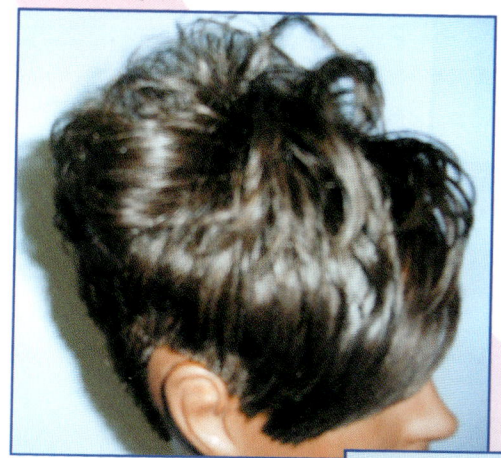

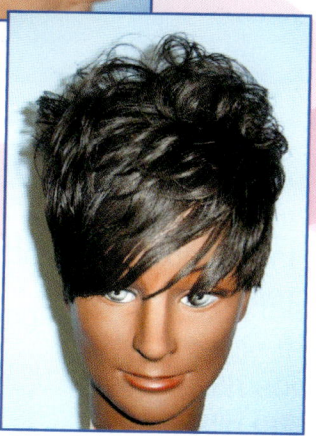

7. A smooth curling effect was achieved. This creates a natural and conservative look.

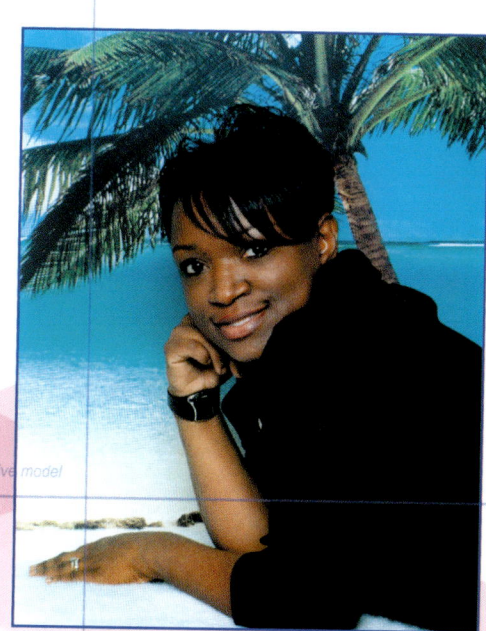

live model

45

Thermal Styling

Basket Weave Design
...continued

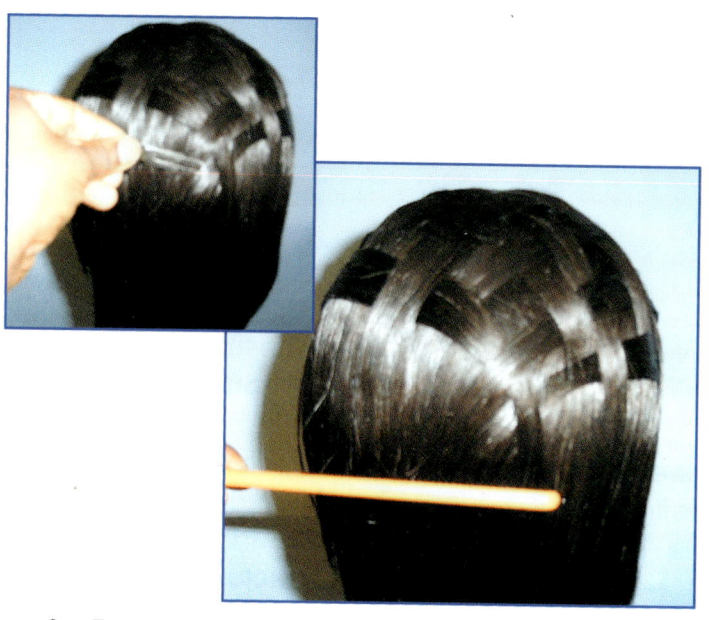

9. Remove clips from hair and blend ends.

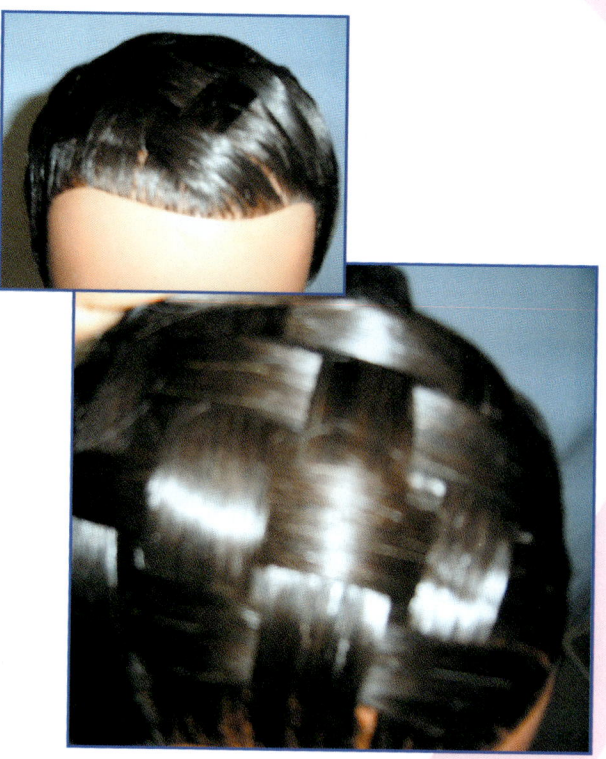

10. A basket weave design is created.

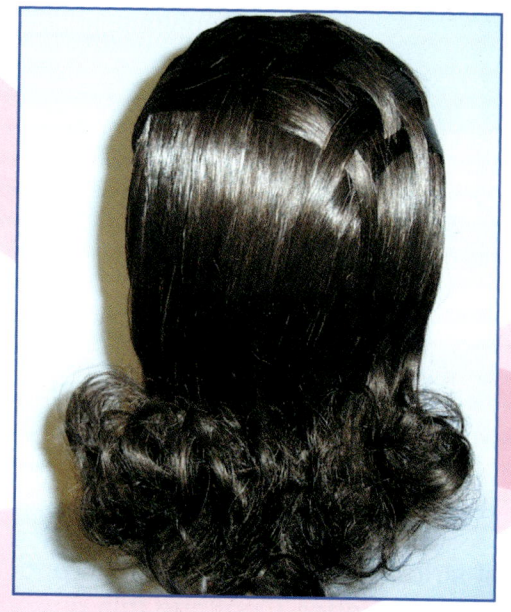
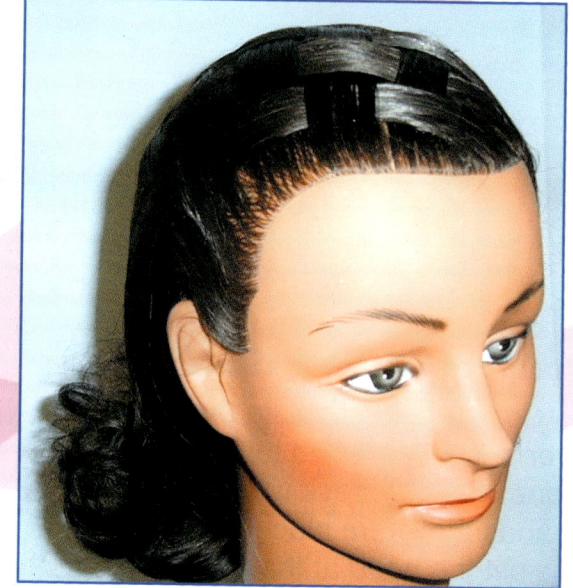

11. Hair is then curled and styled with indentation.

Thermal Styling

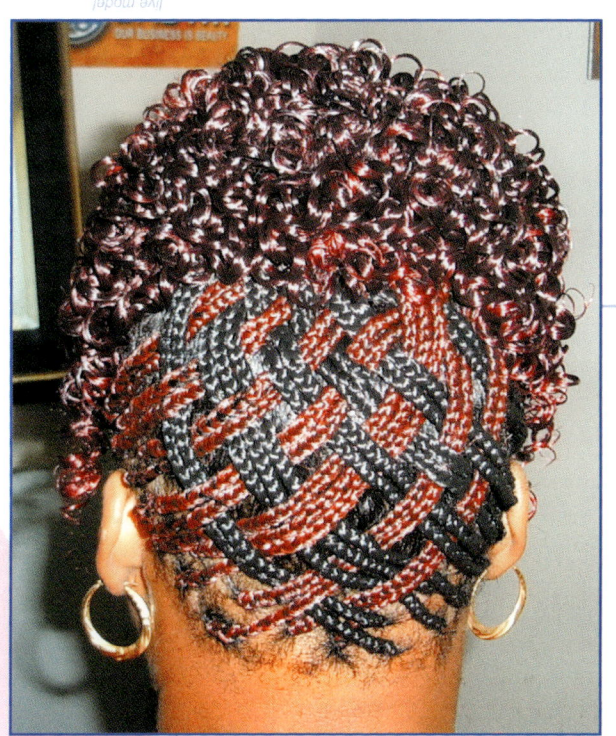

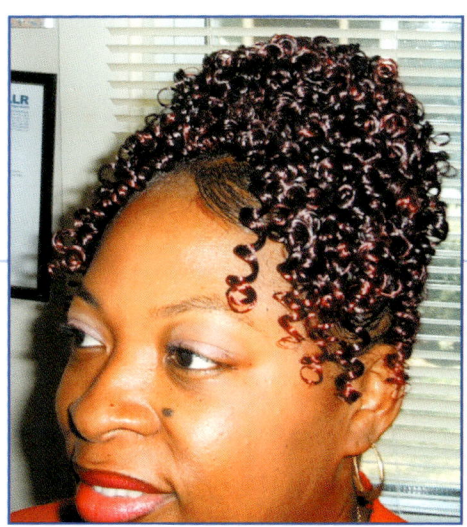

Another variation.

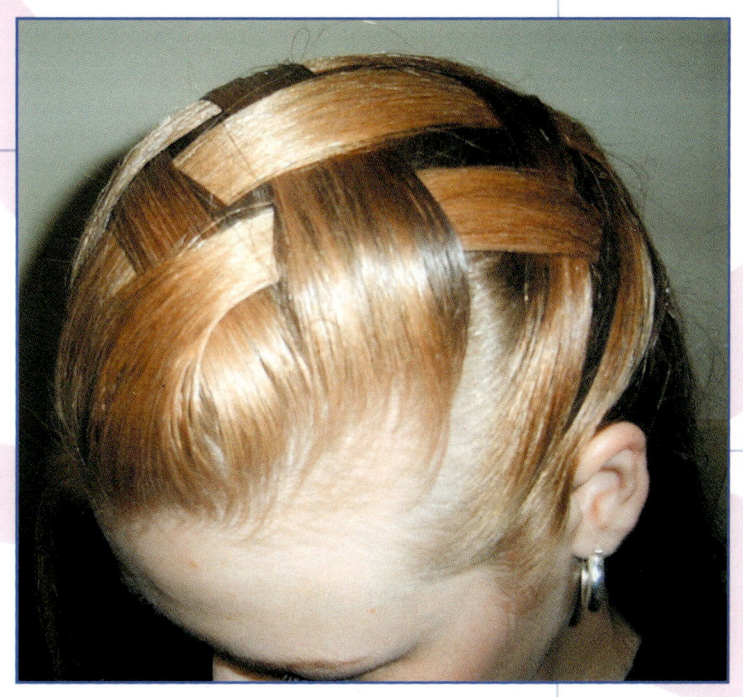

Creativity is everything!

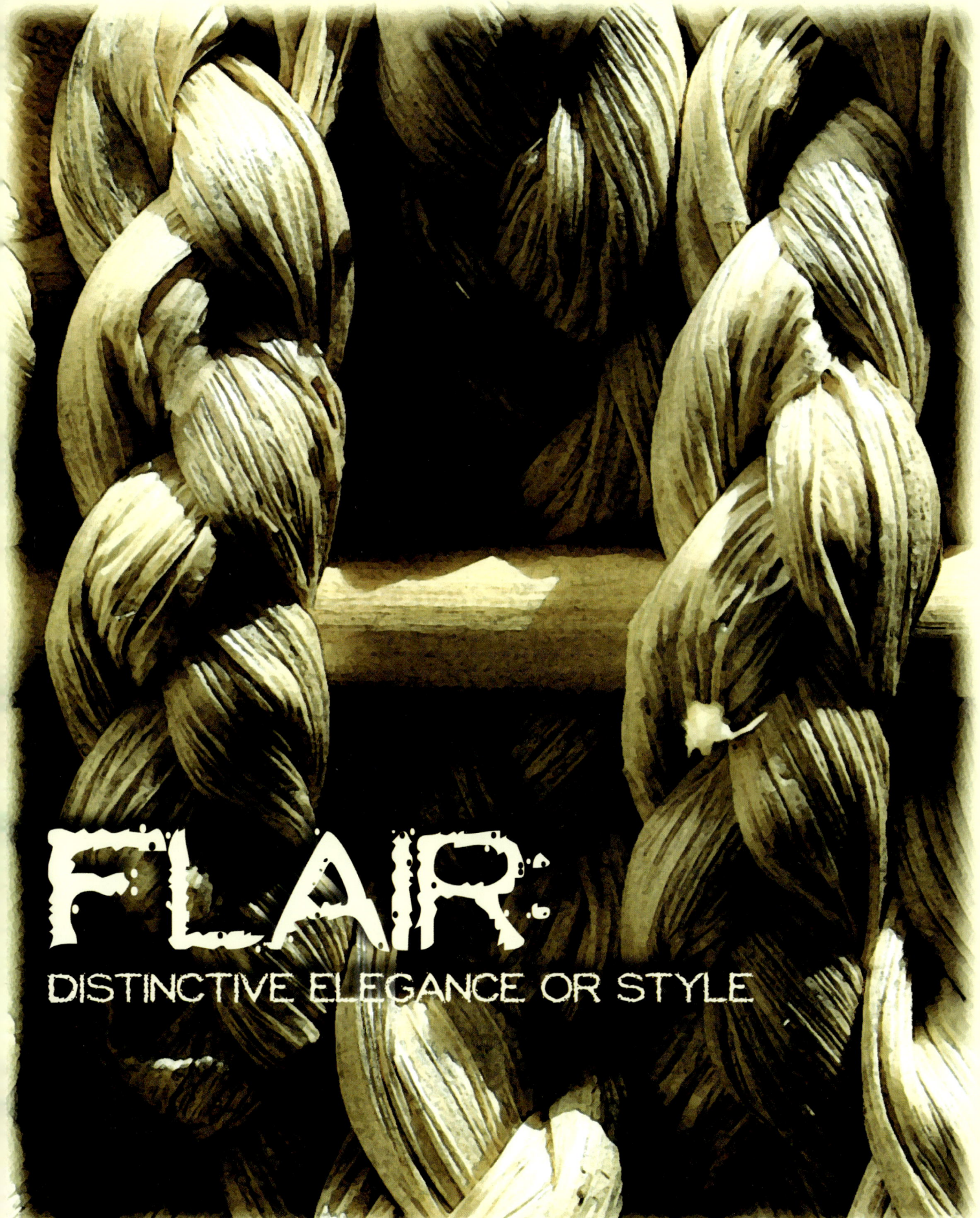

Chapter Five

Braiding and Extensions

Braiding and Extensions

Single Braids
off the scalp braid

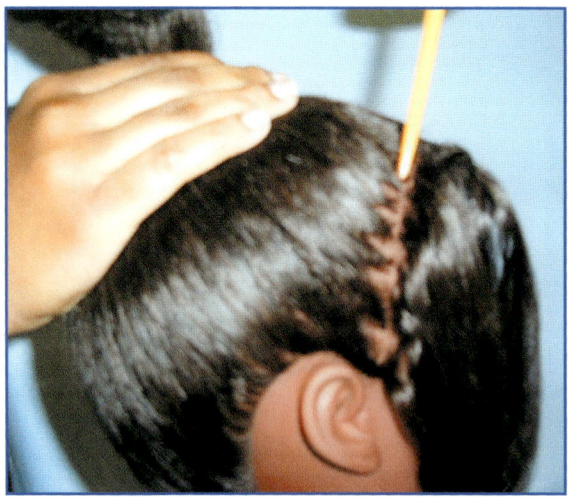

1. Begin by scaling out a one inch diagonal back line from center of forehead to the end of hairline. Place a ponytail in the crown area. Secure ponytail with a rubber band.

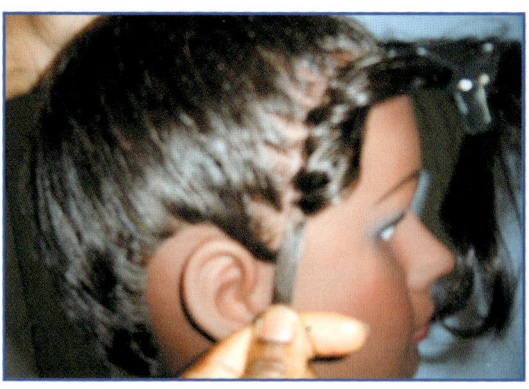

2. The one inch section is used for the off the scalp single braid. Take a small section out from the front hairline.

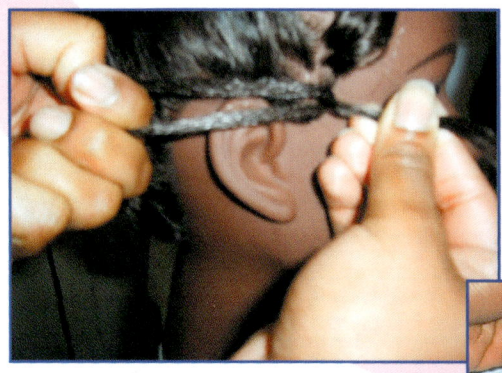

3. Place hair fibers to natural hair. Be sure to keep equal tension.

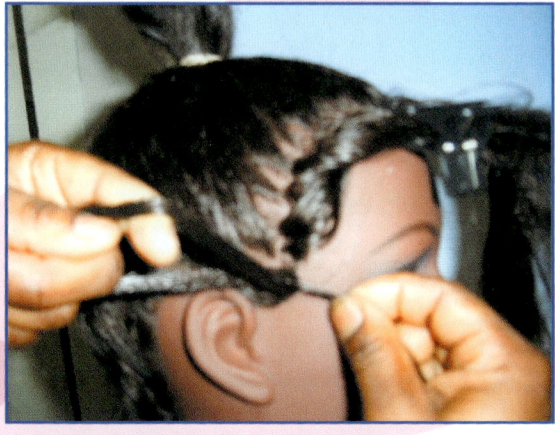

4. Hold the natural hair with tension. Cross the middle hair fibers over the outside hair strand with the left hand.

Braiding and Extensions

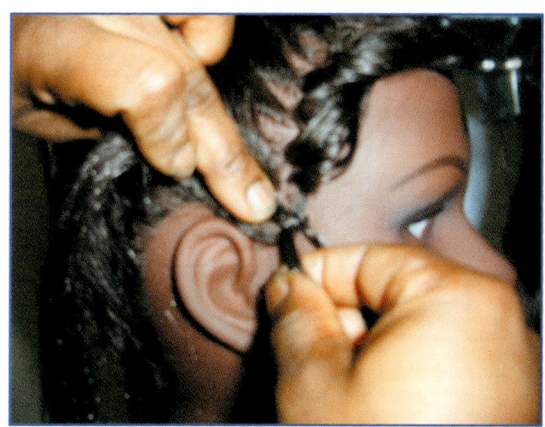

5. Hold left strand with tension. Grasp the middle strand.

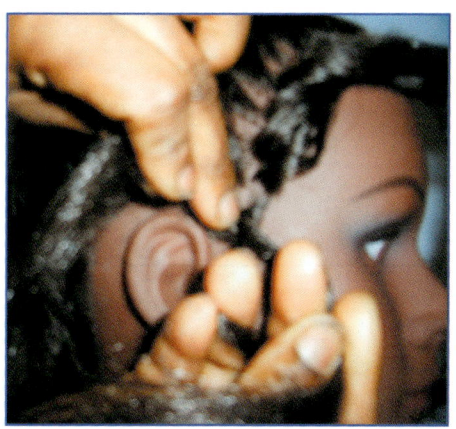

6. While holding the left strand, cross middle strand over right strand.

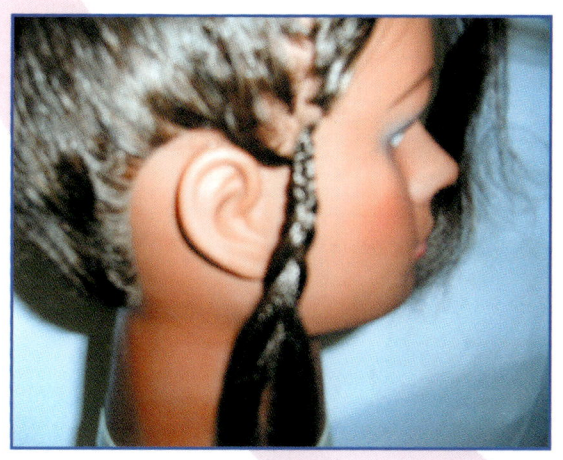

7. Continue this technique, creating an off-the-scalp braid.

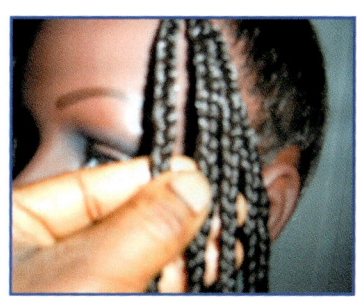

8. Continue to braid down the strand of hair with even tension.

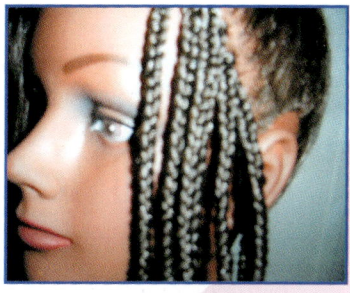

9. The size of the braids are determined by the base of the hair strand.

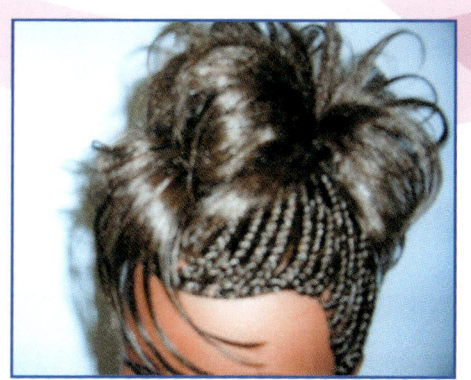

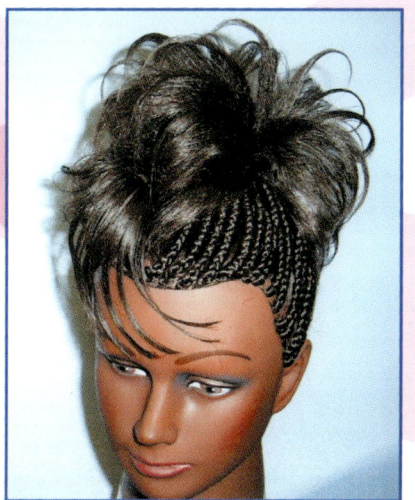

10. Wrap braids around the ponytail and secure with hair pins. Curl ponytail and style with flair.

BraidsBraiding and Extensions

Silky Locks "Dreads"

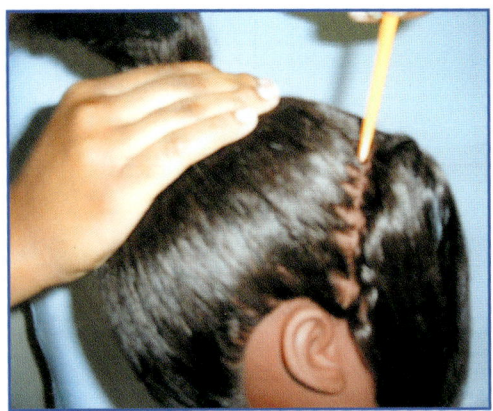
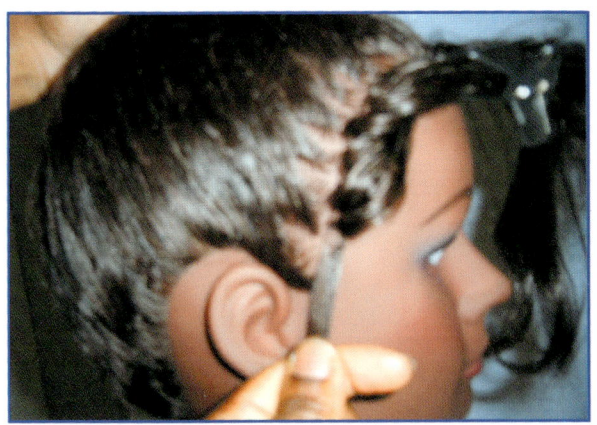

1. Begin by scaling out a one inch diagonal back line from center of forehead to the end of hairline. Place a ponytail in the crown area. Secure ponytail with rubber band.

2. This one inch section is used for the silky locks. Take a small section from hairline.

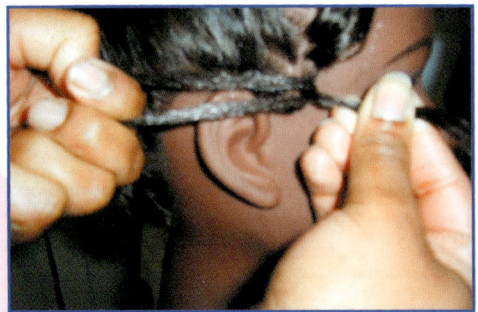

3. Place hair fibers to natural hair. Create a half inch off the scalp braid. This is used for a base to attach additional hair fibers to create a silky lock.

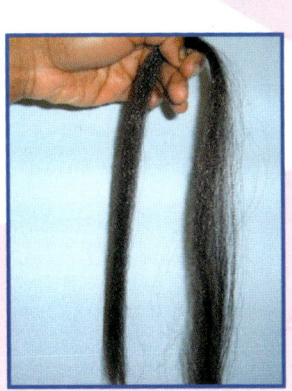
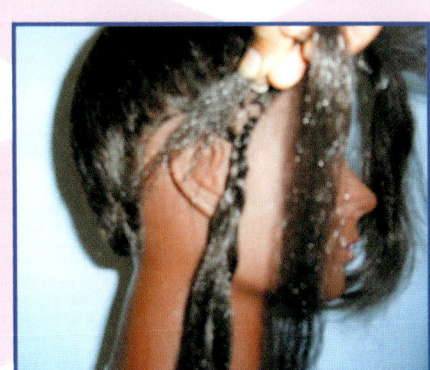
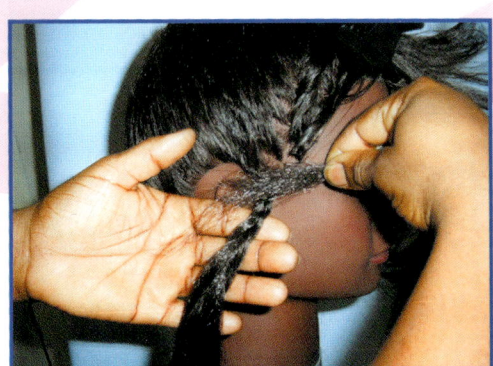

4. Place another piece of hair fibers at the base of the braid.

Braiding and Extensions

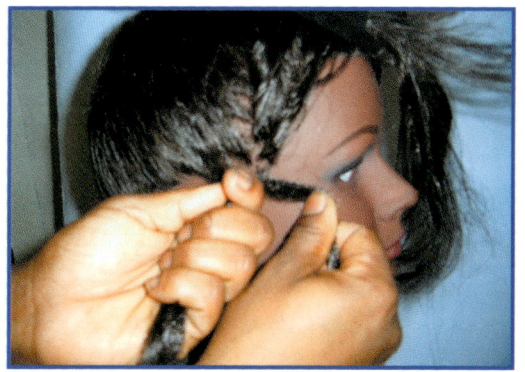 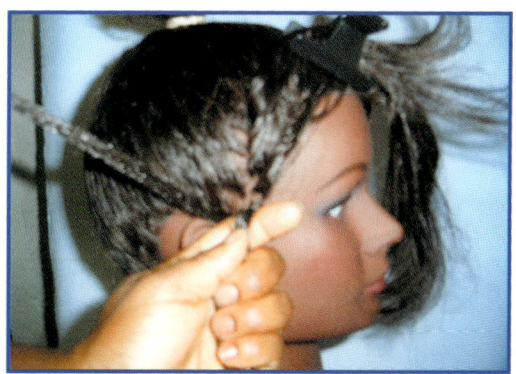

5. Wrap hair fibers around the half inch braid.

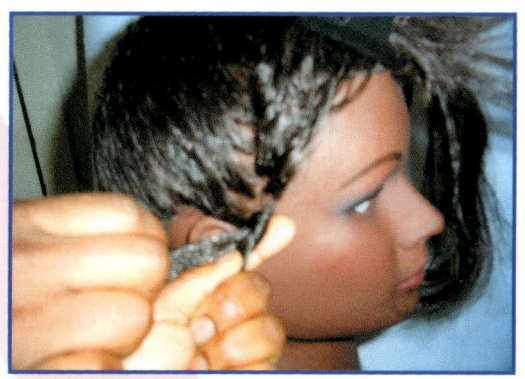 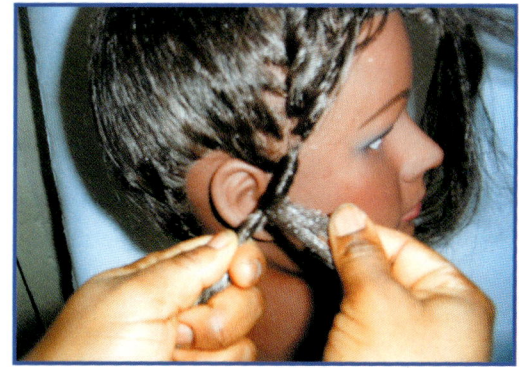

6. Continue to wrap fibers as your work down the strand.

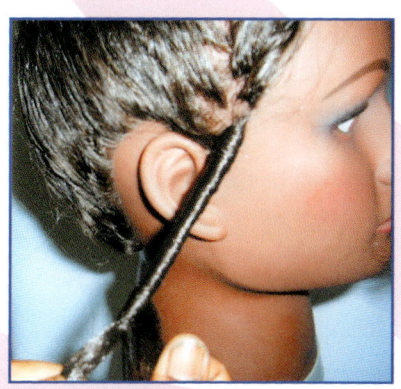 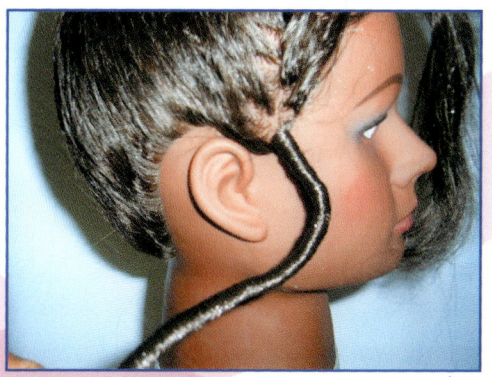

7. Overlap fibers to lock in place. This creates a strong hold so the silky locks will not unravel.

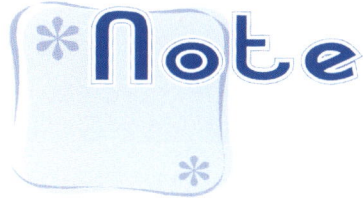

Tension is used throughout both the single braid and silky locks procedures. Keep in mind the movement of finger control will require a great deal of skill.

Braiding and Extensions

Silky Locks "Dreads"
...continued

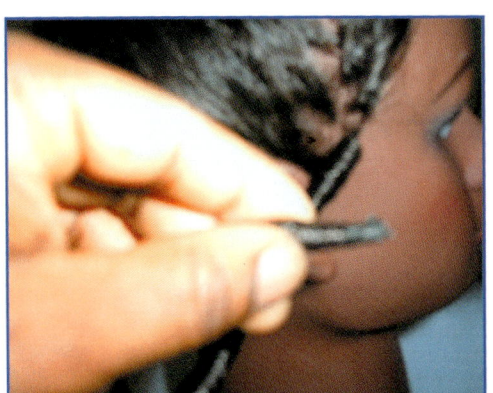

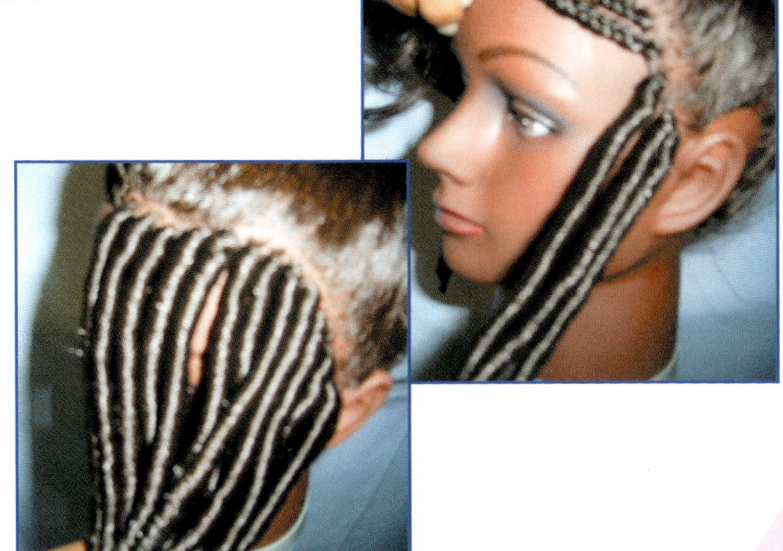

8. Make sure you wrap the hair fibers at least two inches past the natural hair. Burn ends to hold in place.

9. Continue to braid each section a half inch. Use the same technique for the silky locks as shown here.

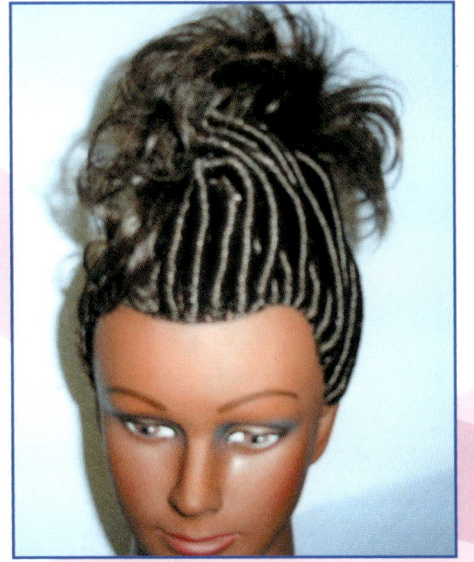

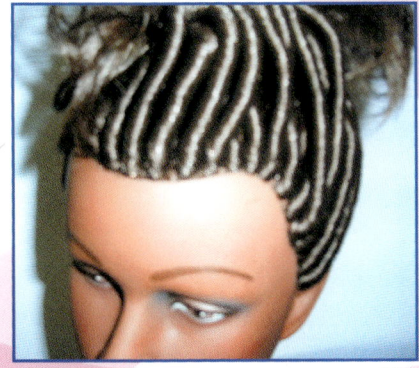

10. Place silky locks around the ponytail and secure in place with hair pins. Curl ponytail and design an intimate look and feel..

Braiding and Extensions

Be Unique!

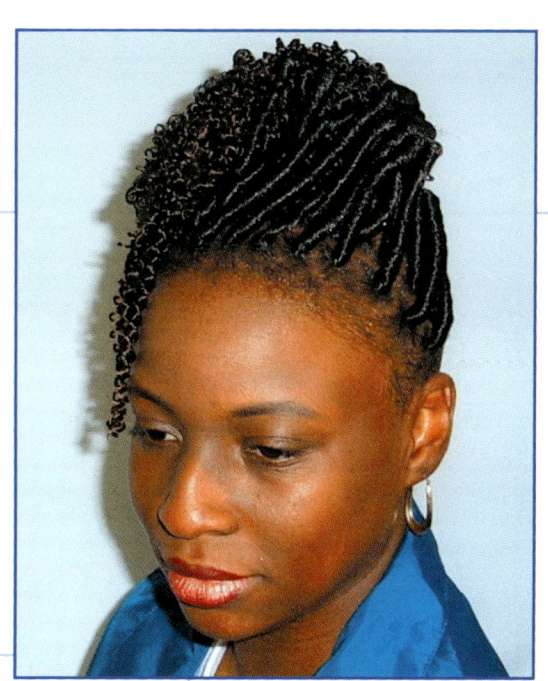

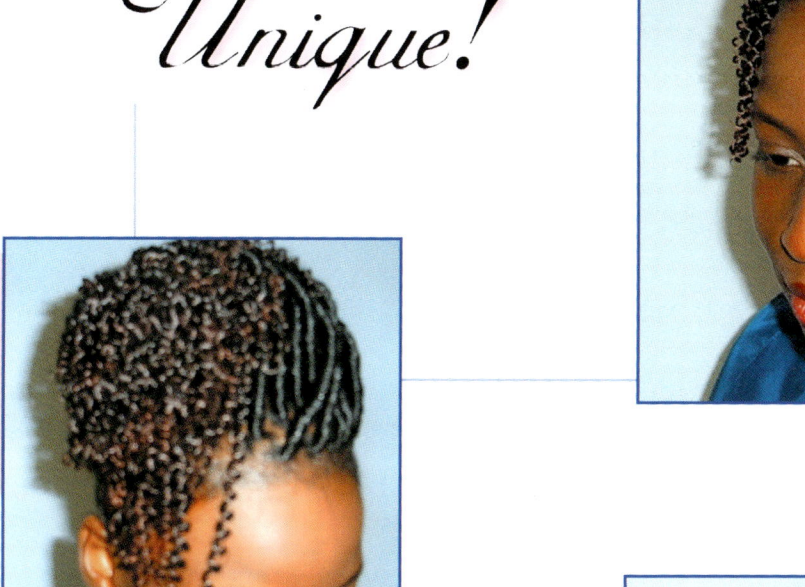

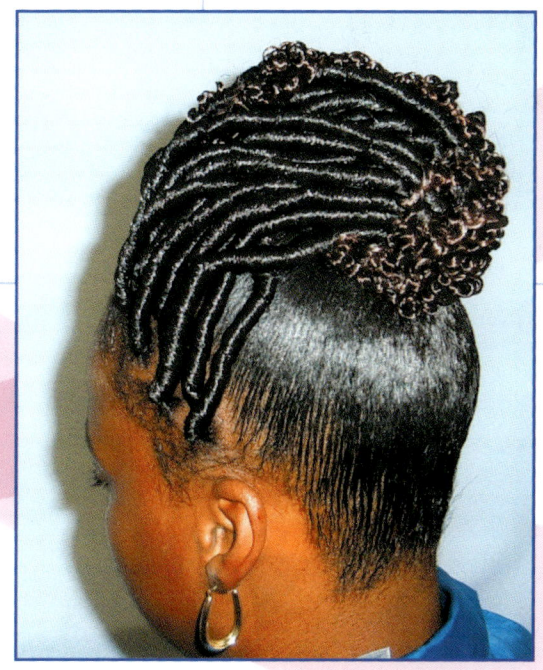

Be Inspired!

57

Braiding and Extensions

Cornrow Braids
on the scalp braid

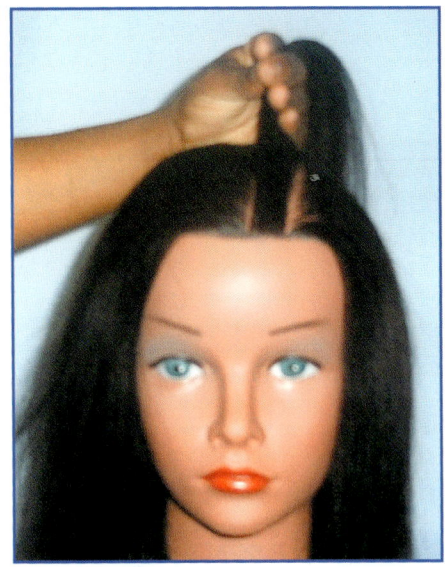

1. Start by parting out a thin vertical section.

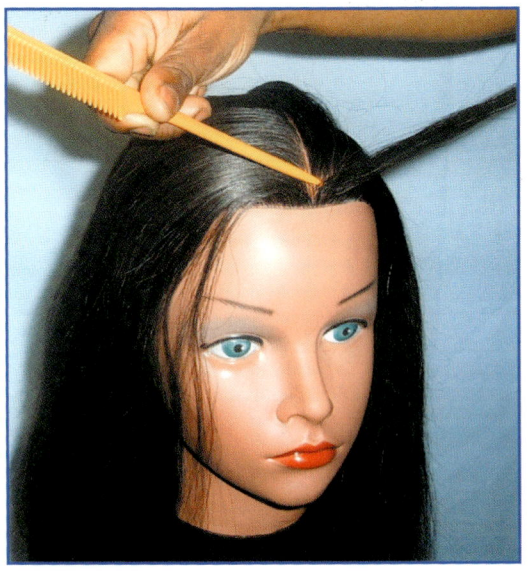

2. Scale out a small section in front of the part.

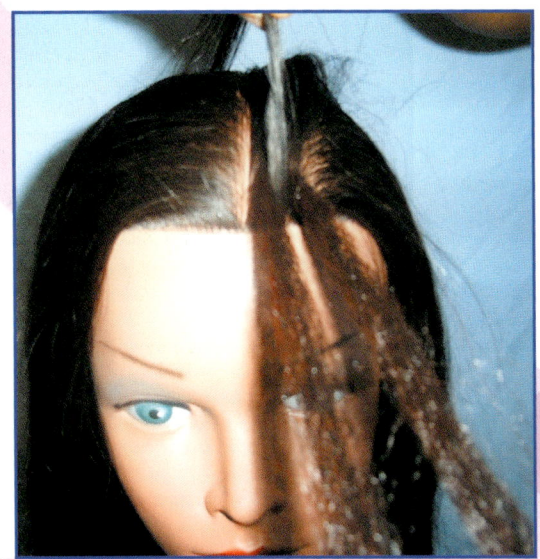

3. Place hair fibers around the small section of the natural hair.

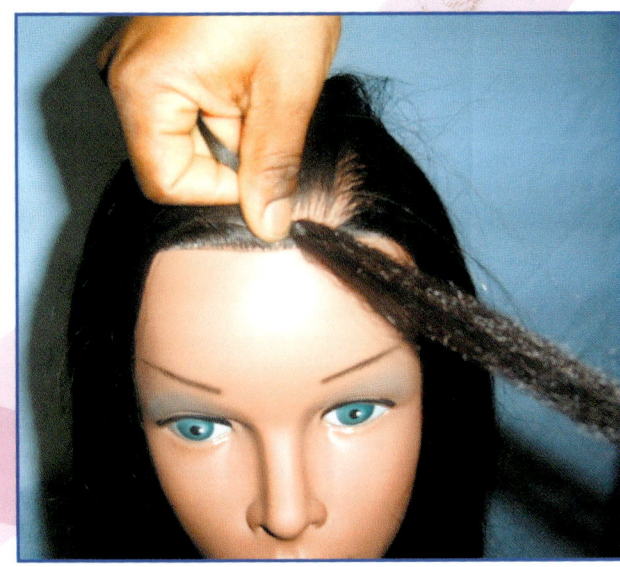

4. Hold the natural hair with your right hand.

Braiding and Extensions

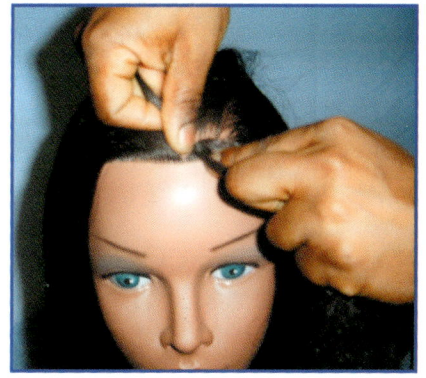
5. Place your index finger between the strands of hair fibers.

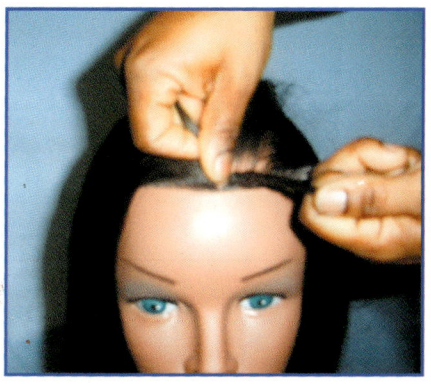
6. Simply turn your left palm up. The left outside strand will cross over the center strand.

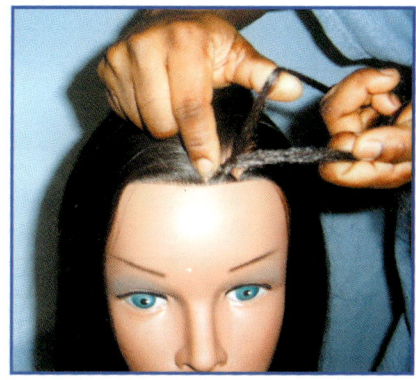
7. Begin to grasp the middle strand with your right hand thumb.

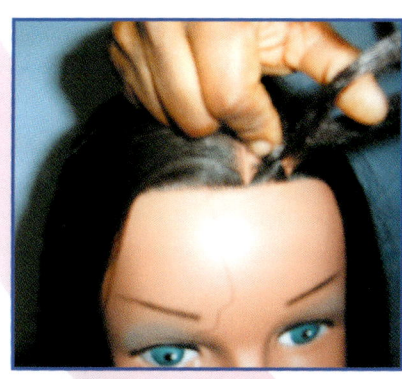
8. Make sure the right index finger continues to hold the natural hair at this point.

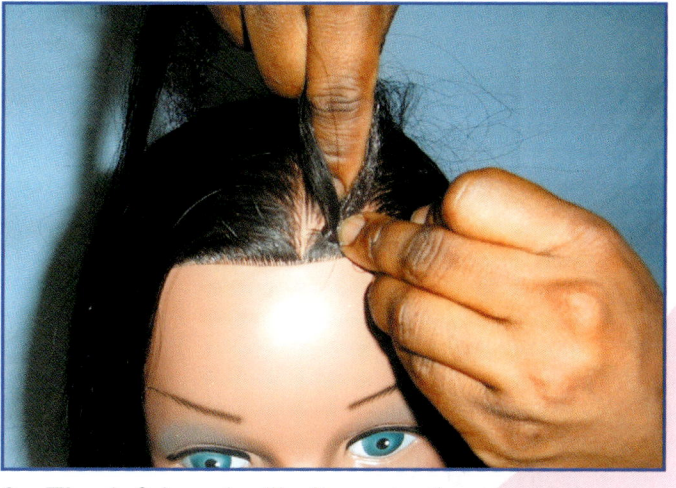
9. The left hand will alternate the same procedure. Hold hair with the left middle finger and turn your right hand crossing the strands from the outer edge to the middle.

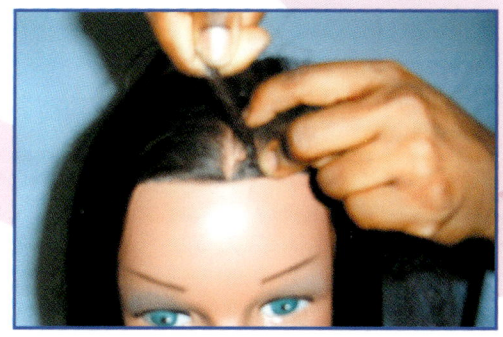
10. Grasp middle strand and continue this technique as you work closely to the scalp.

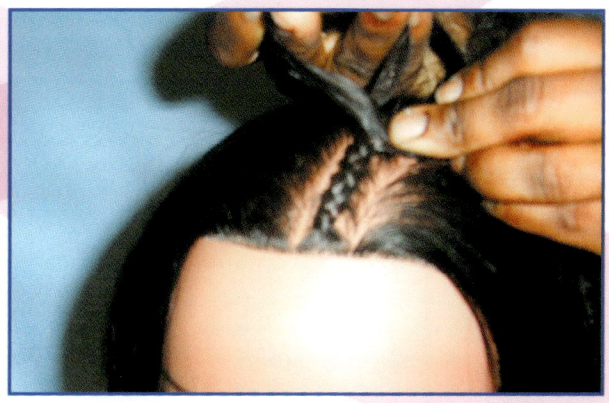
11. Tension is used throughout the technique.

Braiding and Extensions

Cornrow Braids
on the scalp braid ...continued

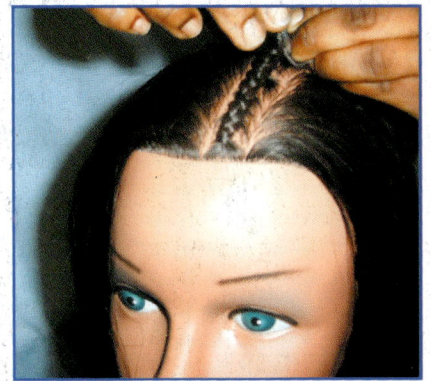

12. A three strand on the scalp braid is created.

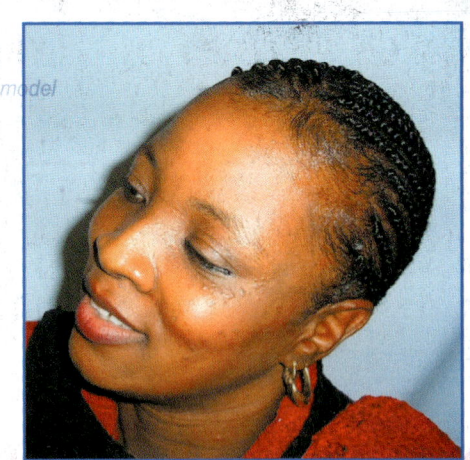

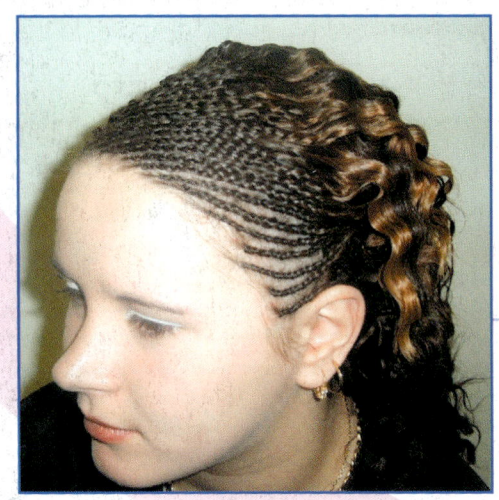

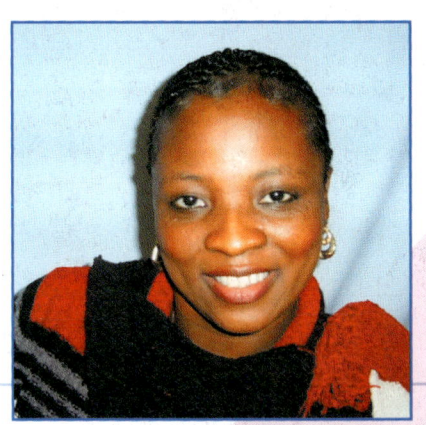

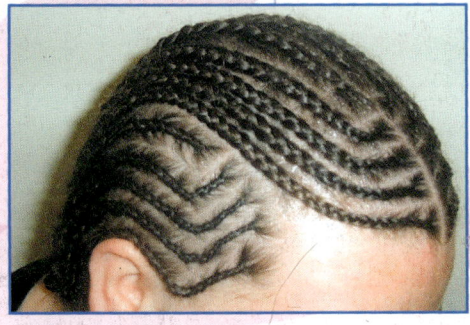

Note
This technique has to have your full attention.
It can be a difficult procedure if you do not have any knowledge of braiding.
Concentration is a must with this design.

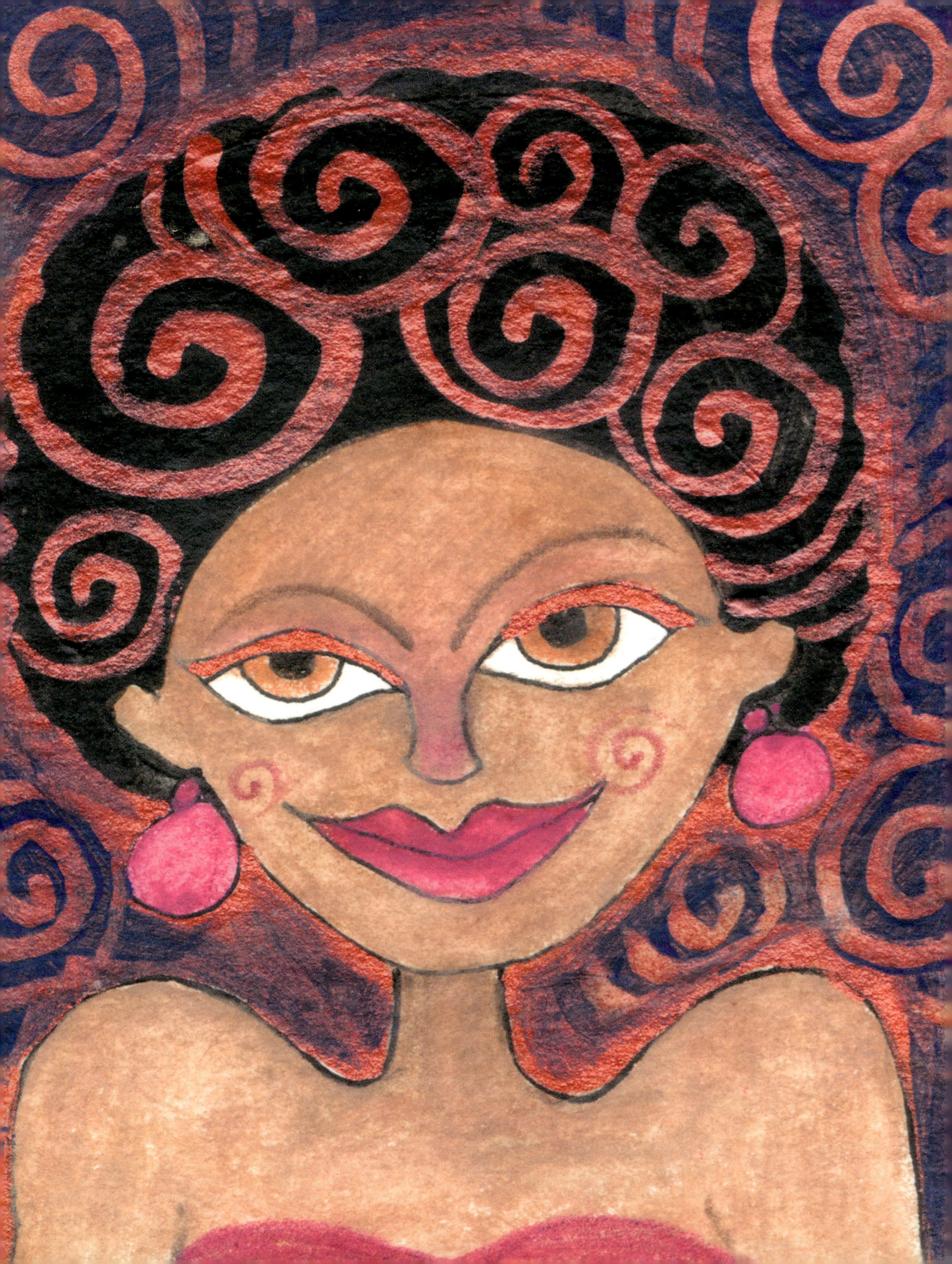

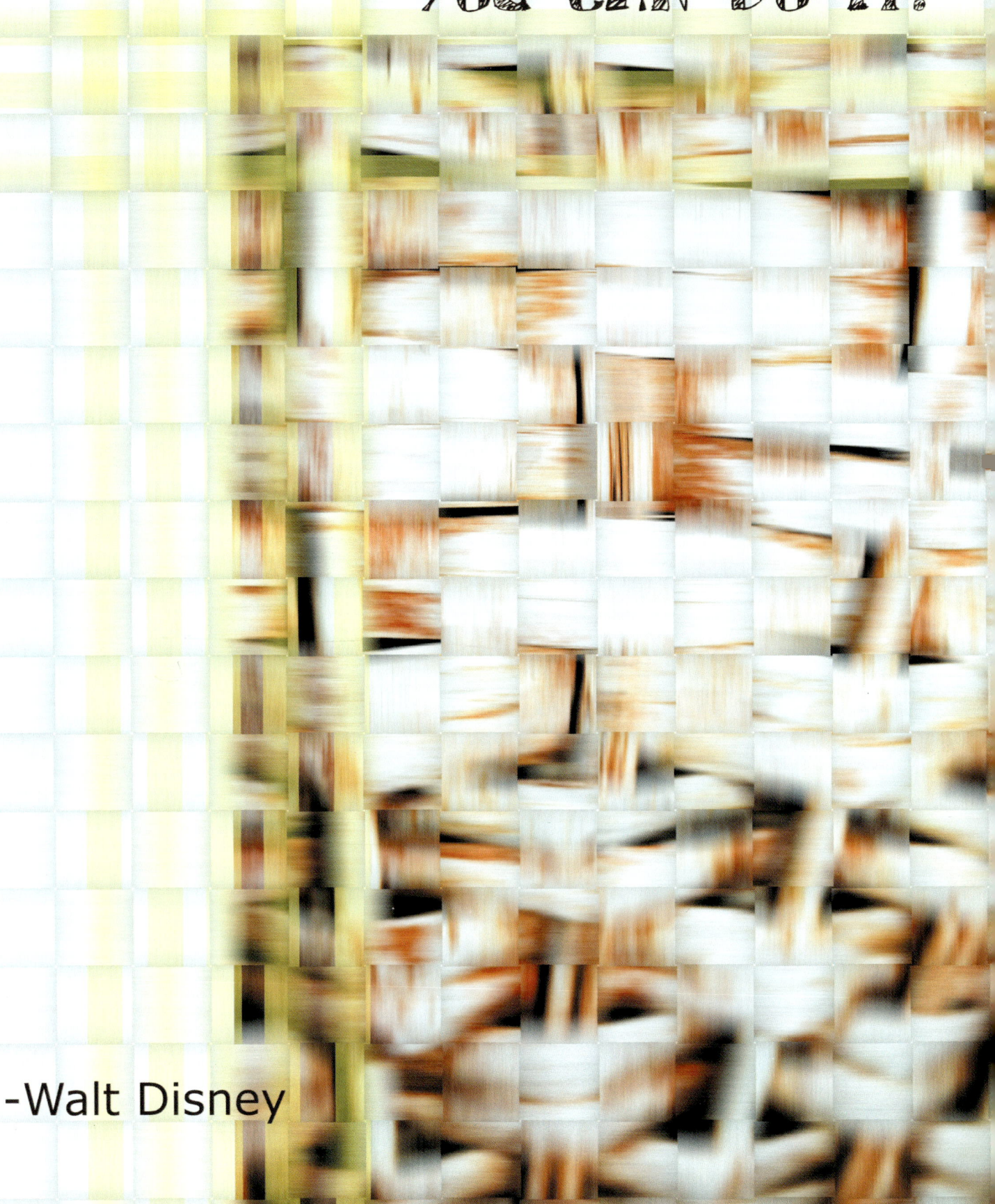

If you can dream it, you can do it.

—Walt Disney

Chapter Six

Weaving

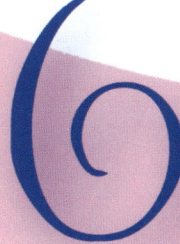

Weaving

Hair Extension
sewing method

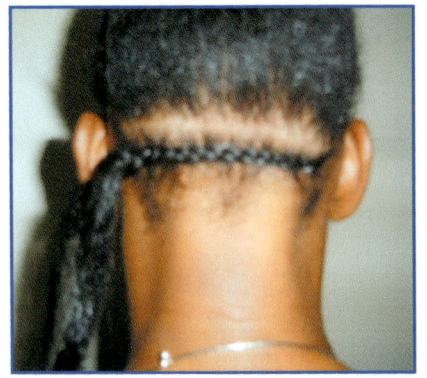 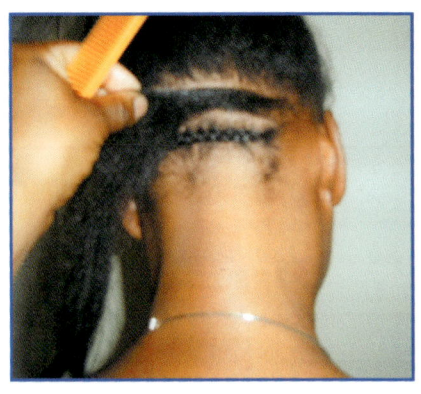 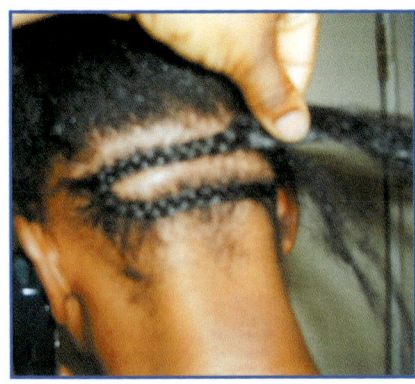

1. Begin by braiding a three strand on the scalp braid. Section out a one inch horizontal part above this braid.

2. Incorporate previous braid to the one inch section above the braid.

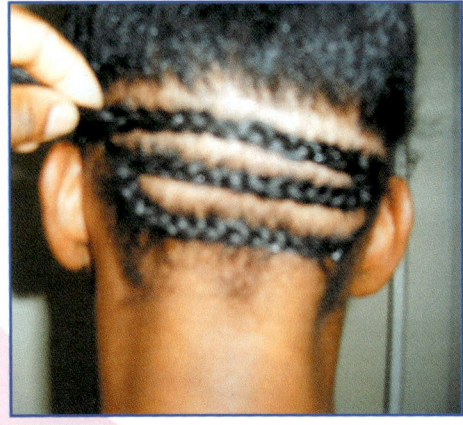 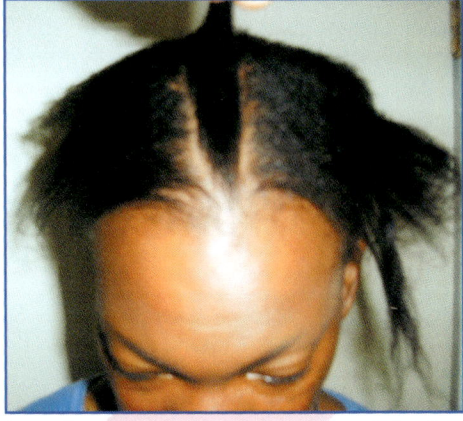

3. Continue to braid in the opposite direction, creating an alternating oblong. Continue this technique up to the crown area.

4. A two inch subsection is molded out in the crown area. This will be used as the finishing touch to this design.

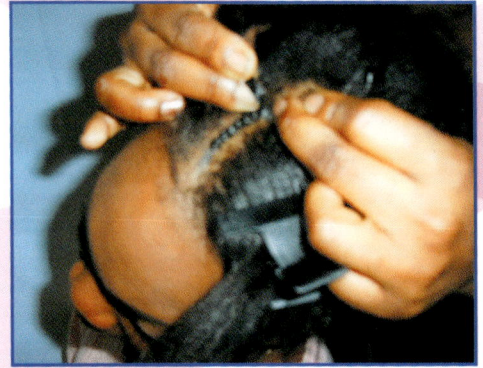 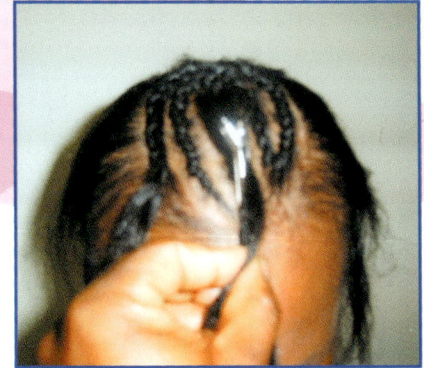

5. Start at the front hairline, creating a circular pattern. Continue to braid until you reach the crown area.

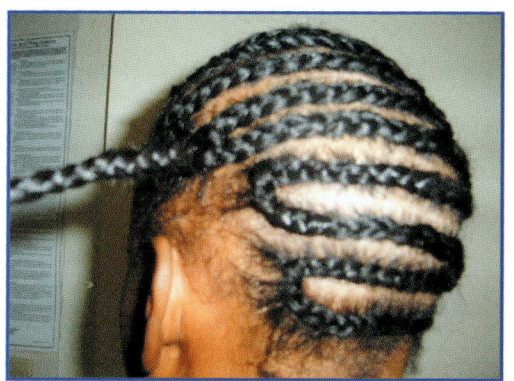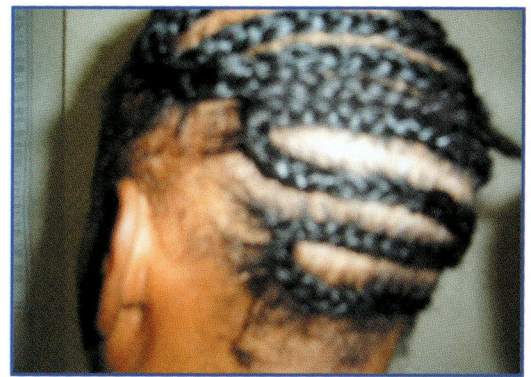

6. Once the entire head is braided, connect the loose braids together. Fold braid between braids and secure with needle and thread to previous braid.

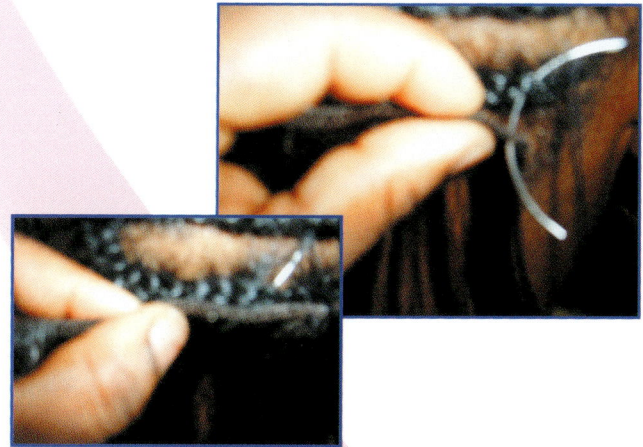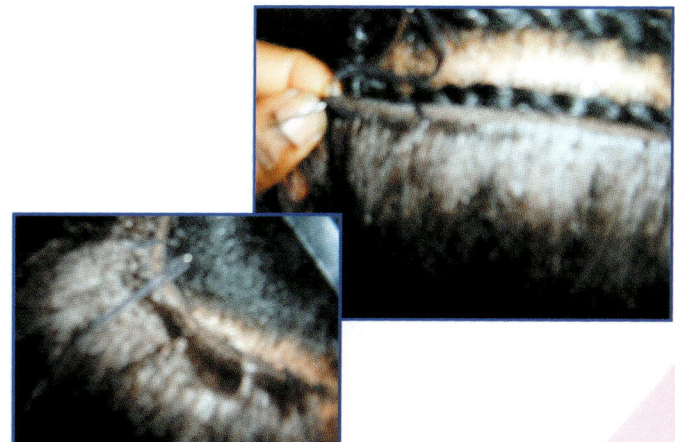

7. Begin to sew the weave onto the braid, starting in the nape area.

8. Continue to attach weave to braids using the sewing method until you reach the subsection in the crown area.

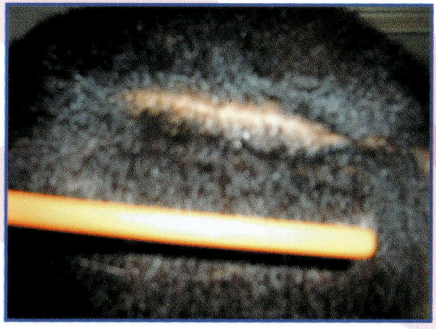

9. The natural hair in the crown area is molded over the weave. This will finish the design.

Weaving

Hair Extension
sewing method ...continued

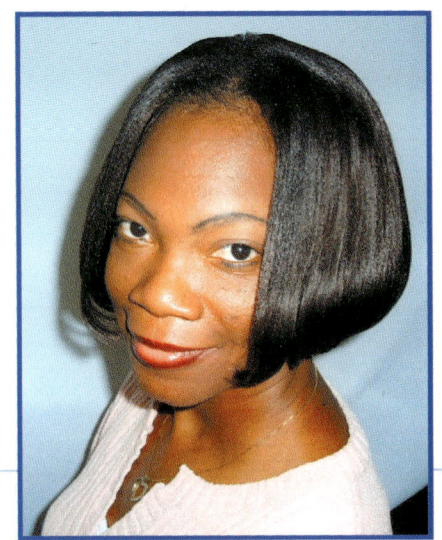
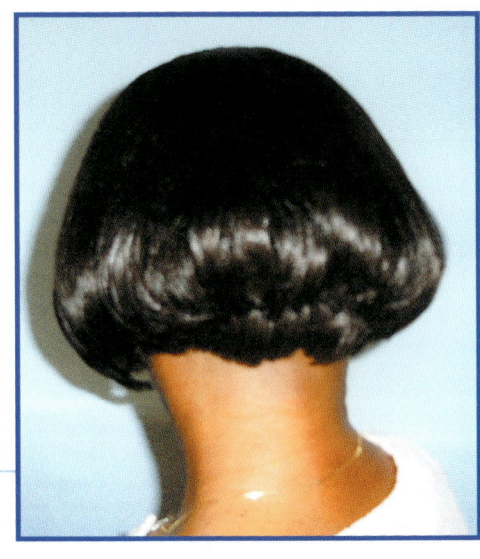

This style was sculpted in a graduated form in the nape area and diagonal on both sides. This creates a softer look for the everyday approach.

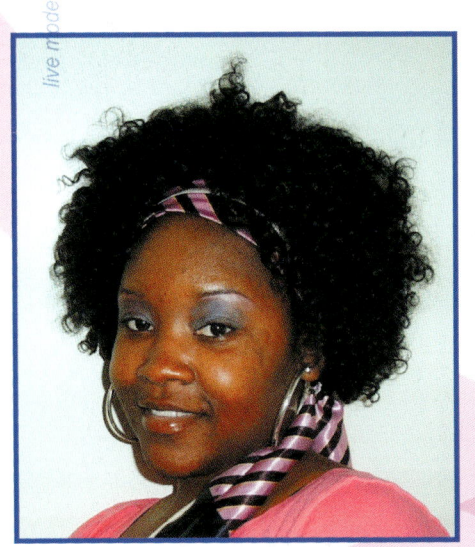
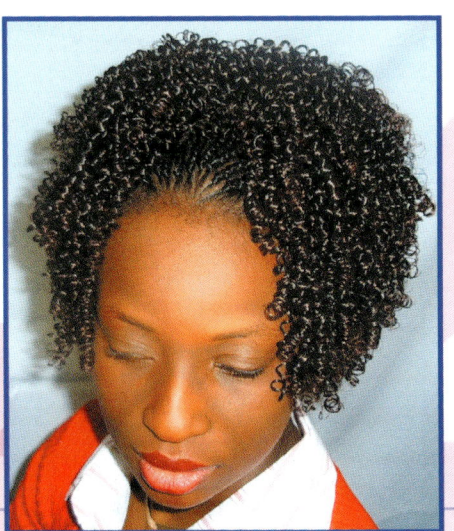
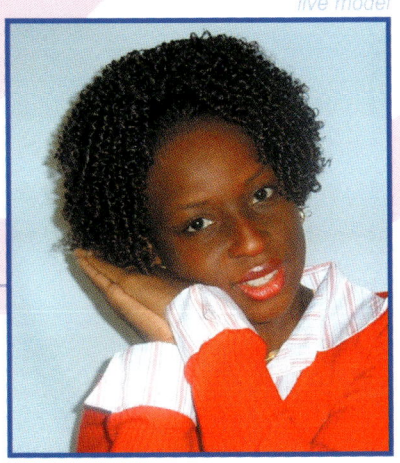

The braiding and sewing technique on pages 64-65 can also be used to achieve the curly full head weave designs.

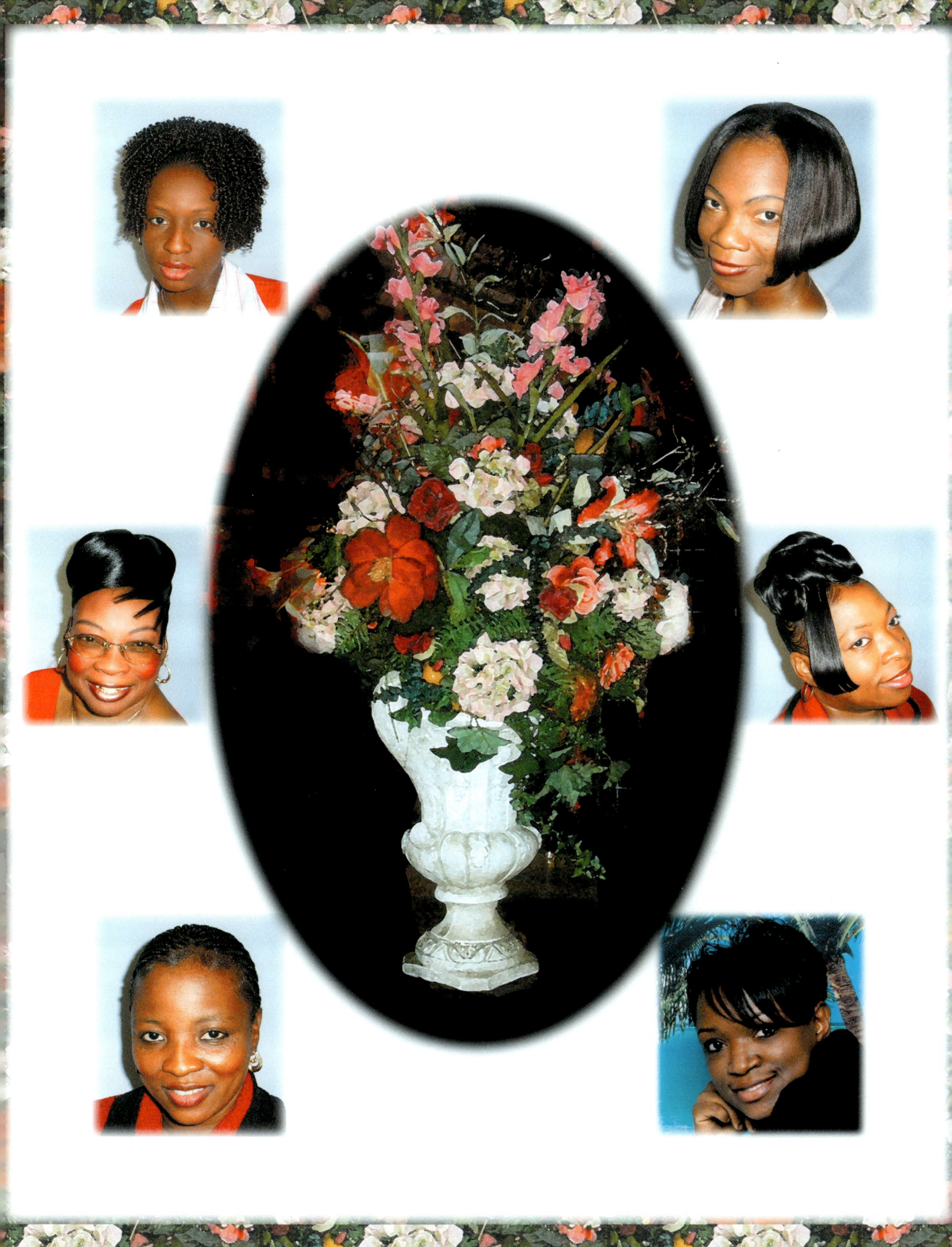

Weaving

Hair Extension
bonding method

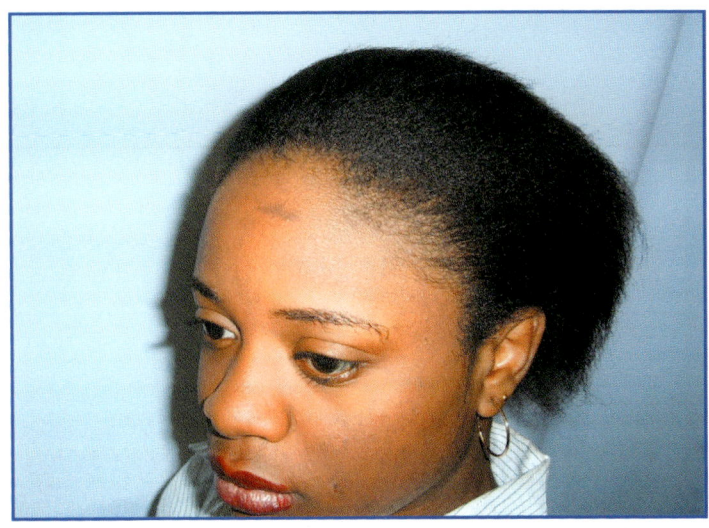

1. Begin by shampooing and blow drying clients natural hair.

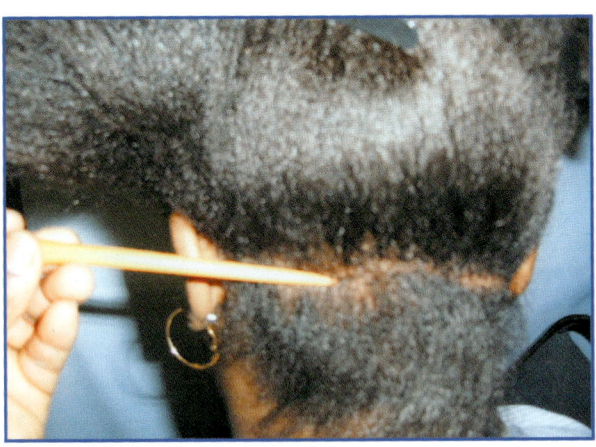

2. Starting in the nape area, begin to carve out a horizontal part. This will give you better control of the hair during the bonding process.

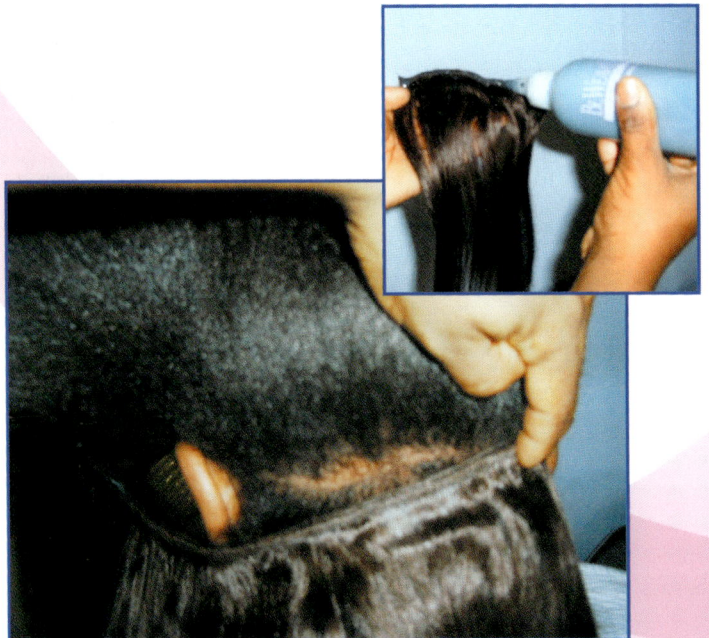

3. Measure and cut weave to match the existing part. Place glue on weave.

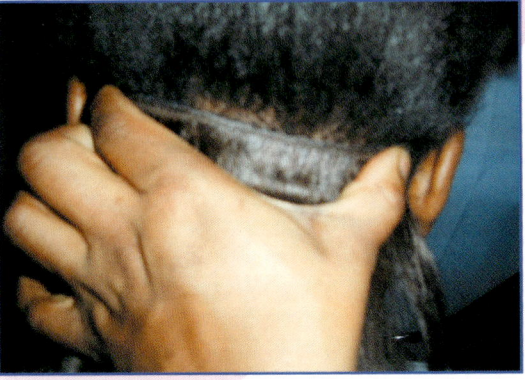

4. Place weave half on and half off the scalp. Begin to blow dry in a rotating back-and-forth fashion.

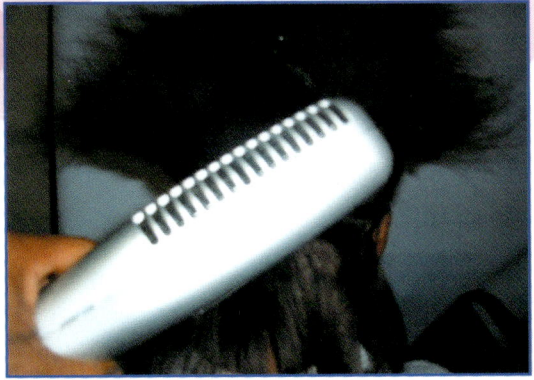

Weaving

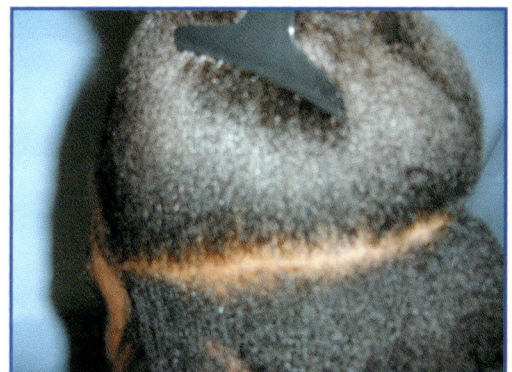 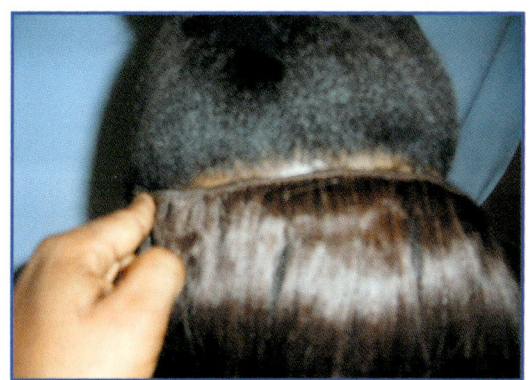

5. Continue to carve out sections and repeat the same technique as you work up towards the crown area. Make sure each section is properly dried.

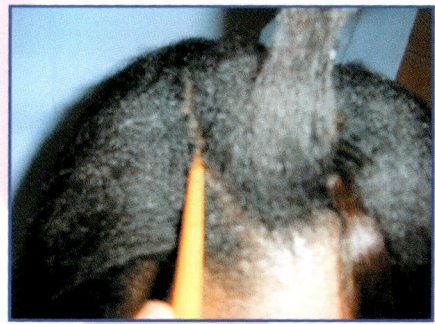 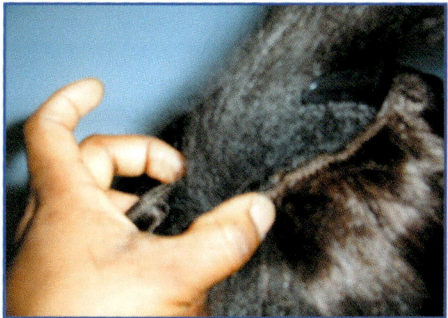 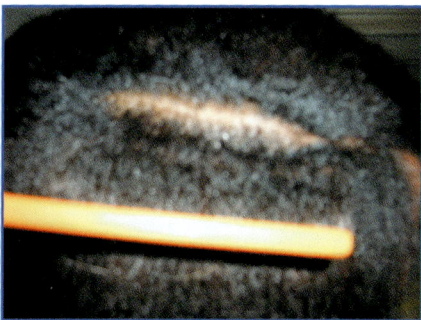

6. Mold out a two inch subsection from the front hairline. This will be used to cover the weave at the end of this design.

7. The last piece of weave is bonded around the two inch subsection.

8. Mold subsection to cover the weave, adding a side part to enhance the design.

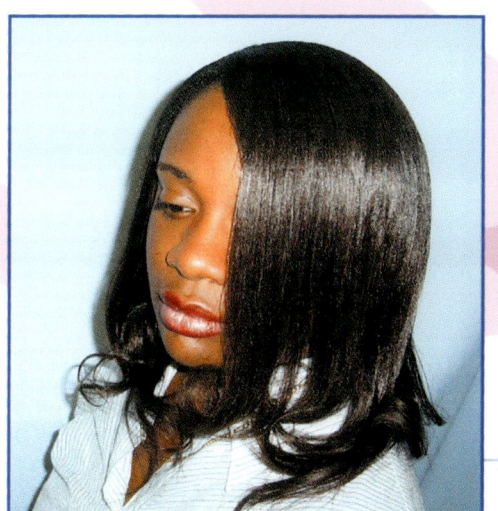 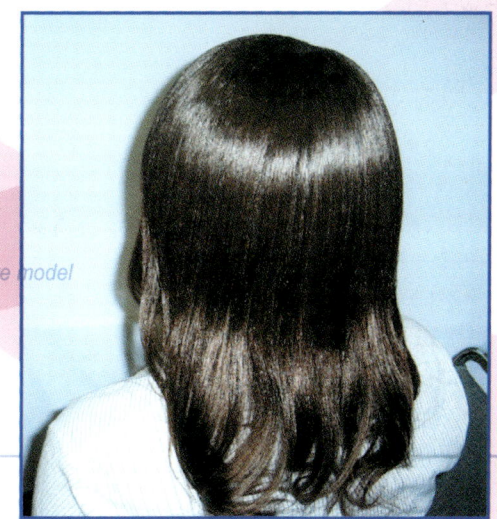

live model

9. A long, fashionable design creates a conservative look.

Weaving

Quick Weave Design

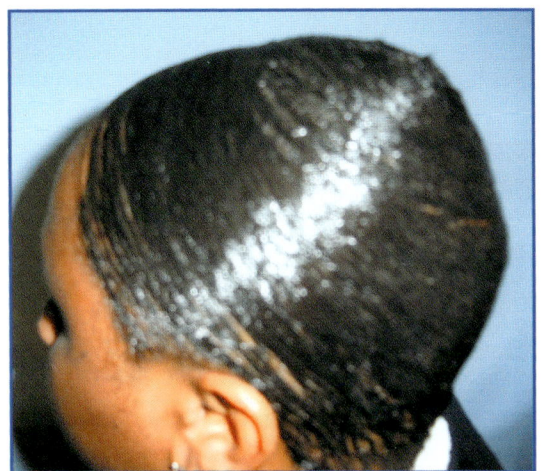

1. Shampoo and then wrap hair. Place gel on top of the wrap.

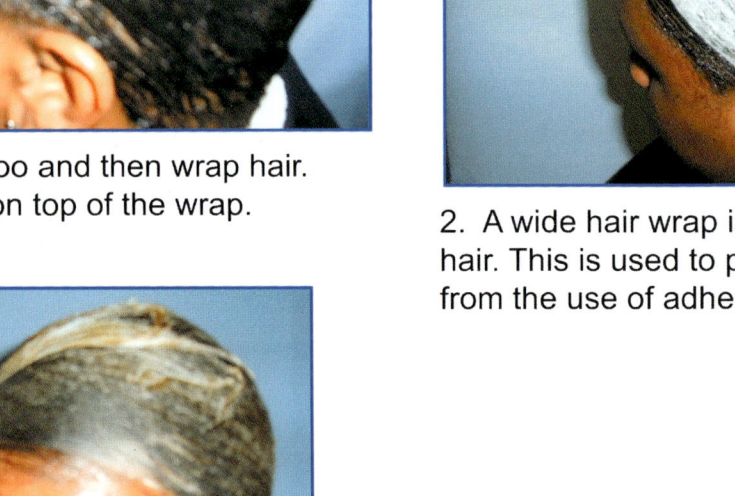

2. A wide hair wrap is then placed on the hair. This is used to protect the natural hair from the use of adhesive.

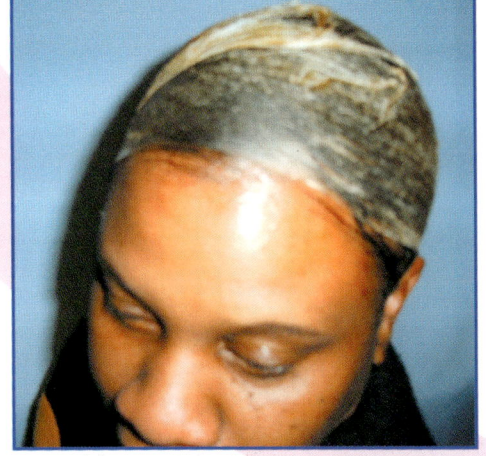

3. The hair is then placed under the drier for thirty to forty-five minutes. This will ensure a complete drying time for the design. A paper maché is the result of this action.

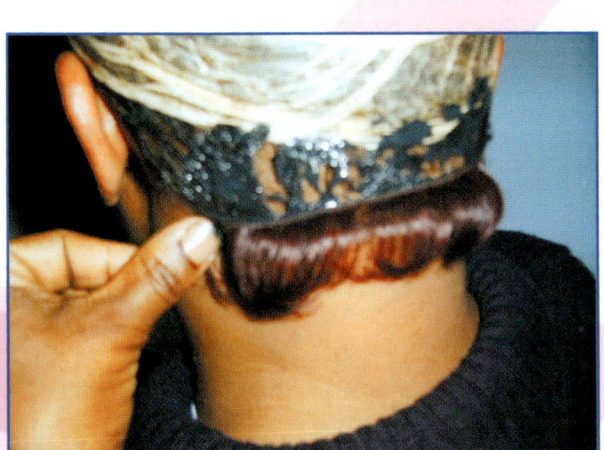

4. Starting at the nape, glue is applied in a circular pattern. Small pieces of hair are then placed on top.

Weaving

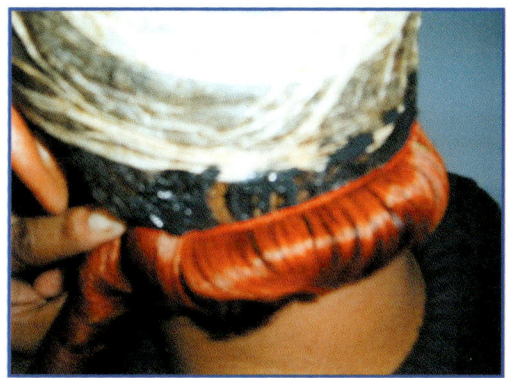
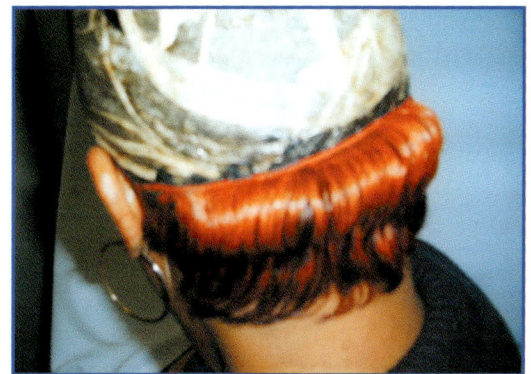

5. Continue to work towards crown area, placing hair one after another and drying as you go along.

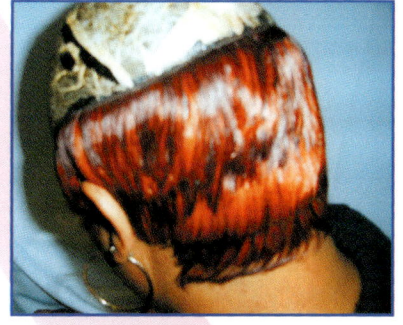
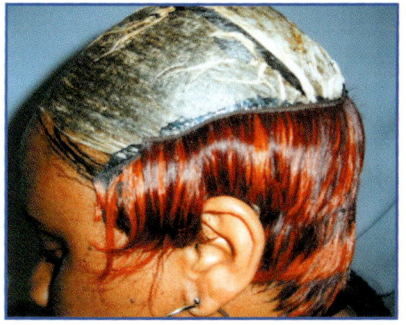
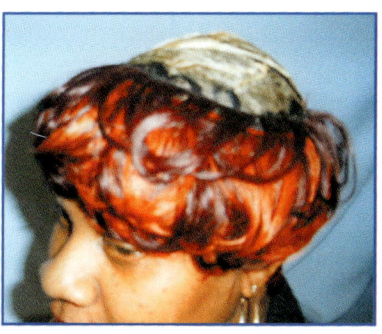

6. This will create a smoother Using a diffuser or curling iron will create a smooth look.

7. Continue to work around the head starting from hairline. Cut and shape as you work.

8. Complete crown in a circular pattern. Shape and trim as desired.

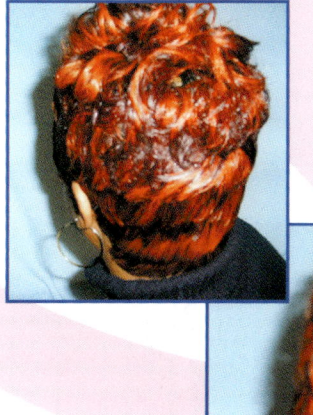
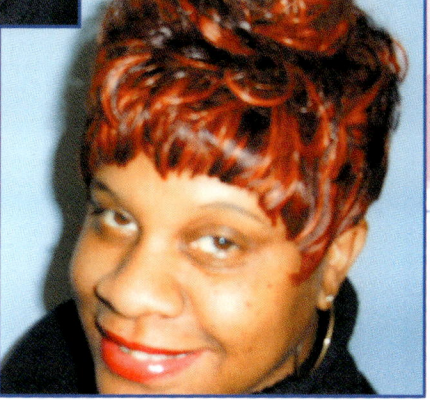
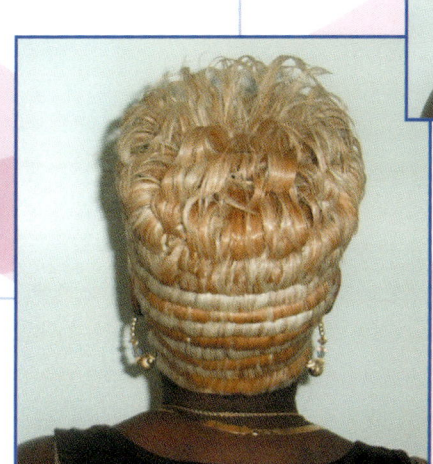

9. Style and curl to finish design.

your
imagination

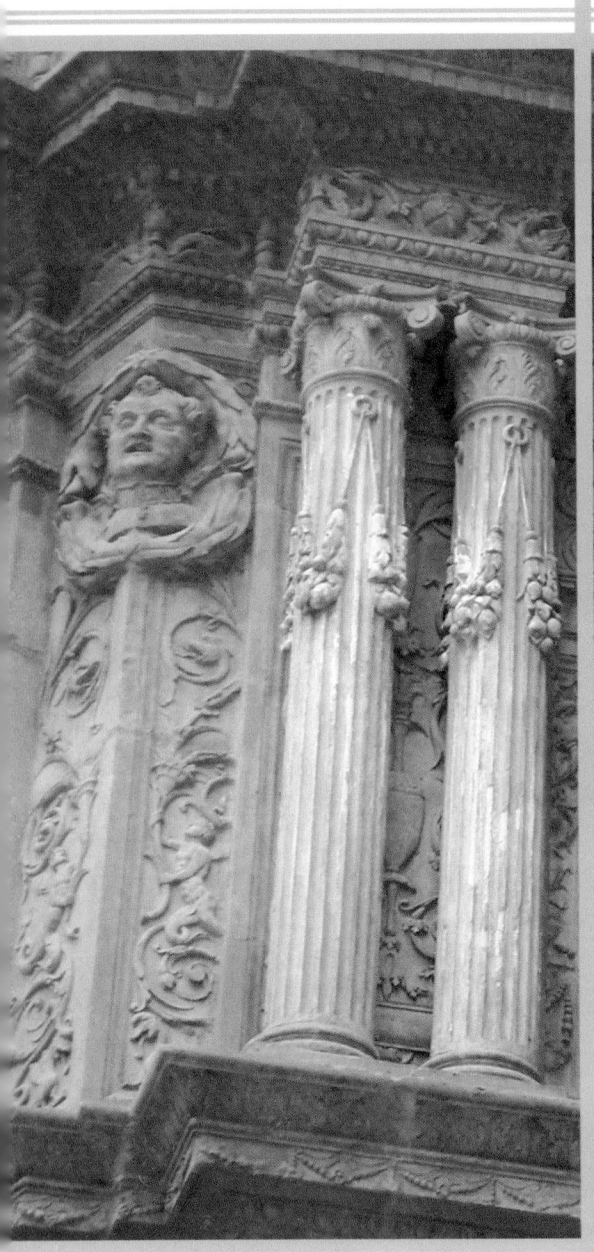
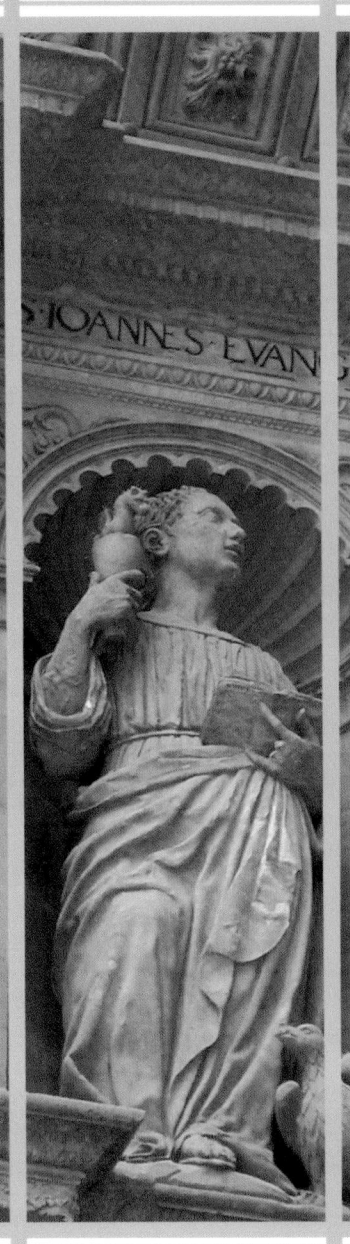
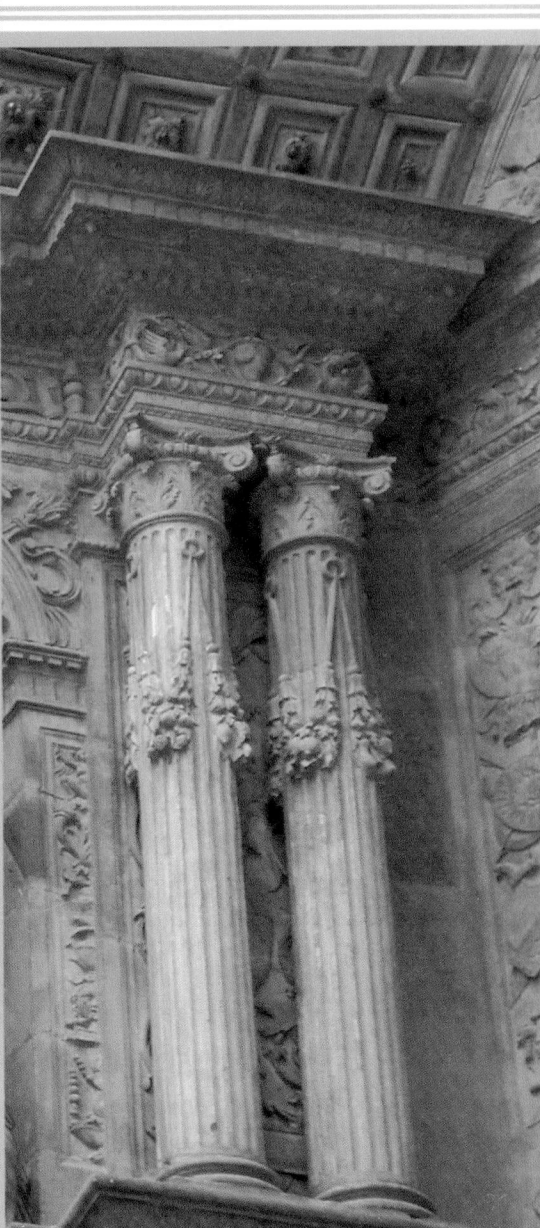

is the
frontier
of your success